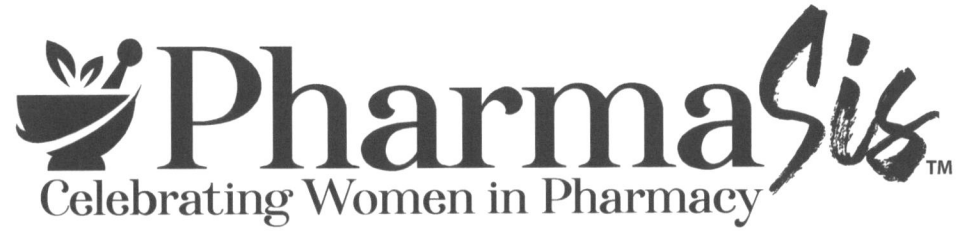

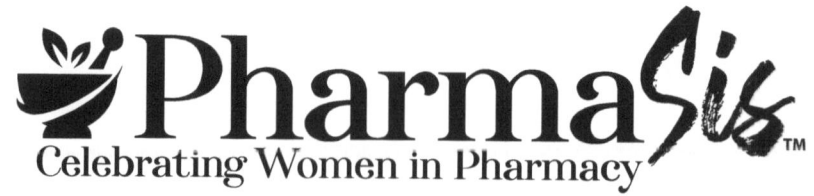

Copyright © 2021 PharmaSis Magazine

All rights reserved. No part of this book may be reproduced or used in any manner without the prior written permission of the copyright owner, except for the use of brief quotations in a book review.

To request permissions, contact the publisher at
www.pharamasismag.com

Printed by PharmaSis Magazine, in the United States of America.

First printing, 2021.

ABOUT THE SUMMER 2021 ISSUE OF PHARMASIS MAGAZINE

This issue of PharmaSis Magazine features women in pharmacy who are dynamic and I want you to know their stories. You will be amazed at their creativity, determination, and their commitment to themselves, their families and their dreams. I am amazed by them!

Check out our first technician feature! You want to read Ms. Keyerra Buckley's story. I am so proud to feature her as our first technician feature and I am so excited to watch her journey!

I'm also proud to introduce our first three contributing authors for PharmaSis Magazine! Each of them was chosen to share their expertise with our readers and they will each write for 4 issues of the magazine! Welcome back to Dr. Christina Fontana (Fall '20) and Dr. Danielle Perrodin (Spring '20) as contributing authors. Both Drs. Fontana and Perrodin were featured pharmacists in 2020 and I am delighted to have them back to share their insights. Welcome also, to Dr. Chinki Bhatia as a contributing author sharing her expertise with our readers.

You can find out more by following PharmaSis Magazine on Facebook and Instagram for updates, videos and encouragement from the featured PharmaSis Magazine women in pharmacy.

You can read more in-depth bios on all of our featured women in pharmacy on the corresponding issue link on the website: www.PharmaSisMag.com.

Be sure to visit the PharmaSis Marketplace on the website, where you can connect to any woman that has been featured in the PharmaSis Magazine to collaborate.

Thank you for celebrating with the PharmaSis community of women!

Celebrating and Inspiring Women in Pharmacy to Build a Life and Career of Their Dreams…

Executive Editor in Chief
Dr. Jerrica Dodd

Creative Director Shannon S. G. Jarrett - Speak Beautiful
Cover Photographer Tessa Swarthout - Tessa Marie Studios
Cover Fashion Stylist Tijuana Faison - Design Faze Boutique
Cover Hair Stylist - Alicia Igess - Urban Tangles Salon
Cover Makeup Artist - Sydney King

PharmaSisMag.com

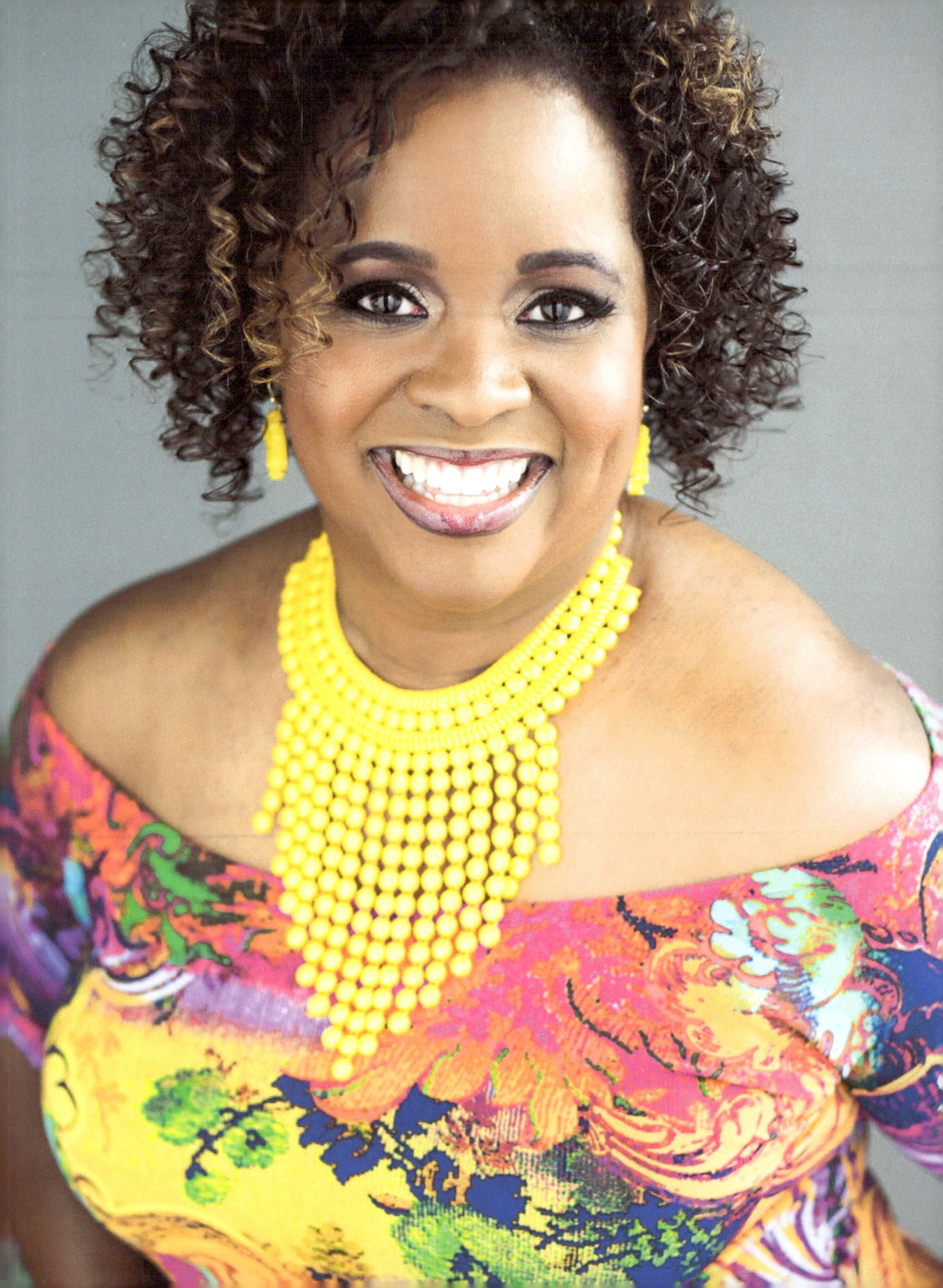

WELCOME TO THE SUMMER 2021 ISSUE OF PHARMASIS MAGAZINE

Welcome to PharmaSis Magazine, where the goal is to celebrate women in pharmacy and share their stories and wisdom. These amazing women are to be celebrated for their courage, brilliance, beauty and passion.

Until about 3 years ago, I thought my story was that I had had brain surgery. People's eyes were wide when I dropped that fact in conversation. What I realized was that, my story was not that I had brain surgery; my story was that as I child I adopted a performance based view of my value and worthiness and it set me up to be a "pro" at people pleasing as an adult. I thought as long as I did what was expected of me and did whatever I could to make others happy, life was great! Well, it took my health for me to understand that I had never prioritized my wants, wishes, dreams and desires. My brain surgery and my subsequent health challenges have continued to remind me that I have to take care of myself or I will have an empty cup from which to pour. Now, I have built a business serving coaching clients and patients, I have traveled for pleasure and business and live in cities that I LOVE, and I have built and continue to be a part of communities that feed my soul! My dreams became urgent and I continue to build them!!

PharmaSis Magazine exists to be a platform where women in pharmacy can share, encourage, inspire and see themselves as the leader of their lives, businesses and careers!

As our world is still in the midst of a global pandemic and we see so many things constantly change around us, I welcome the opportunity to share our featured women in pharmacy and their stories.

Again, Welcome to PharmaSis Magazine!

Jerrica

Dr. Jerrica Dodd
Founder/Executive Editor, PharmaSis Magazine
Founder/CEO, Your Pharmacy Advocate
PharmD, Florida A&M Univ. 1998
MS, Pharmacy Administration, The Ohio State Univ. 2000
MS, Applied Pharmacoeconomics, Univ. of Florida 2012

FROM THE EDITOR

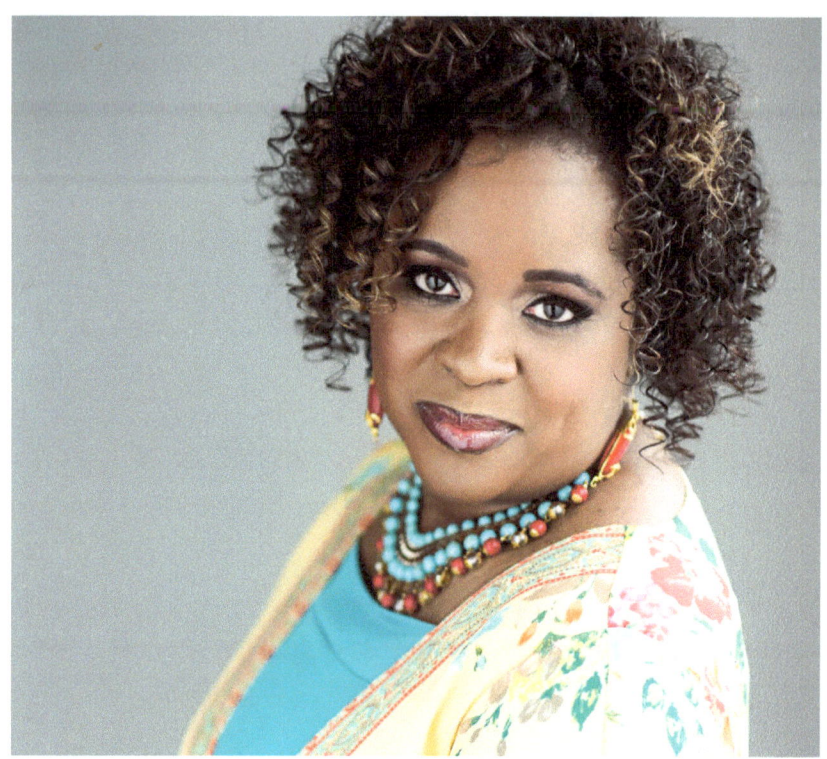

The Summer of 2021 has been unbelievable…while we are still experiencing the coronavirus and any new curve ball it has thrown our world, we are learning and navigating our new normal for our world and our own lives. I have made some tremendous changes in my life as I continue to build my dream and I write this letter from a new place in my dream to live and work from anywhere in the world. So, this issue is being published from Brentwood (Nashville), TN, which has been my first stop since leaving Marietta (Atlanta), GA.

Living life in color and stereo and encouraging women in pharmacy to do the same…

INSIDE THIS ISSUE

on the cover

Reconnecting to Your Heart to Transform Your Business
Dr. Christina Fontana
8

Living Life Unapologetically
Dr. Megan Freeland
10

How the 5 Love Languages Could Make Us Better Pharmacists
Dr. Megan Freeland
16

Everything in Our Country is Refundable but False Information
Dr. Mansi Shah
25

Style Matters
Dr. Danielle Perrodin
52

5 Invigorating Ayurvedic Drinks that Pharmacists can Endorse for Diabetic Patients!
Dr. Chinki Bhatia
60

Putting Health Back in Healthcare
Dr. Mansi Shah
26

The Power of Resilience
Dr. Kristine Mason Cline
32

The Fulfilled Pharmacist
Lisa King, RPH
38

Living Life Fearlessly
Dr. Ani Rostomyan
46

Helping Women Thrive
Dr. Marina Buksov
54

Contributing Author Spotlight:
Meet Chinki Bhatia
56

TECHNICIAN SPOTLIGHT:
Showing Up Fearlessly
Keyerrá Michelle Buckley
18

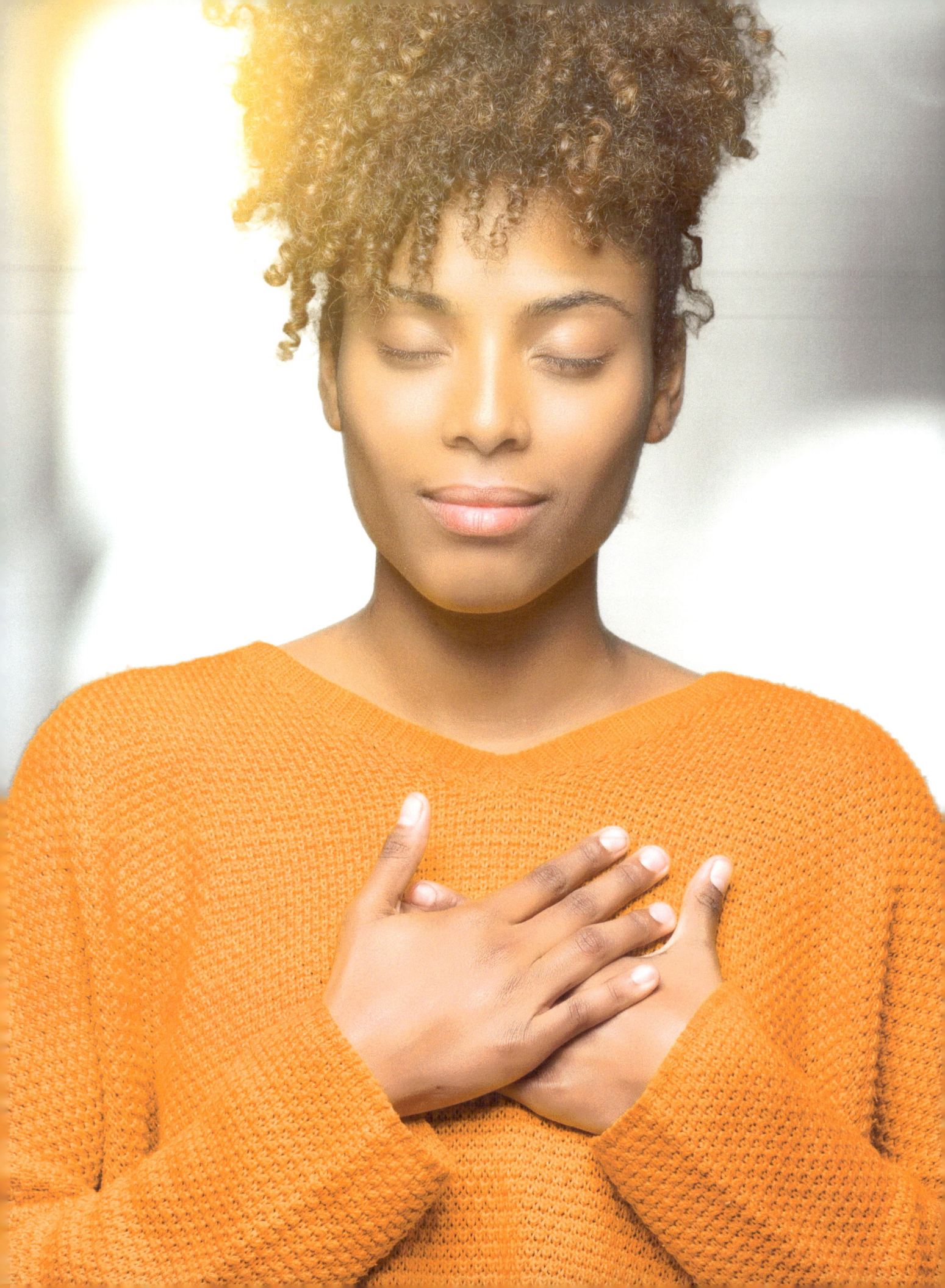

COVER STORY

Reconnecting to Your Heart to Transform Your Business

Written by: Dr. Christina Fontana, *Contributing Author*

In my rapid transformation coaching business, I coach visionary pharmacists looking to make a bigger impact out in the world. They've been in pharmacy (retail, hospital, academia, etc) but they have this gut feeling that there is more they can do to influence their patients. Can you relate?

What I've found in my 9 years of coaching is that the most powerful way to accelerate the path to greater levels of income and impact comes down to one word – transformation. Transformation involves deprogramming old beliefs and stories along with releasing certain blocks so that you can show up as the most authentic version of you. This allows you to access more power, confidence, and self-expression as you tap into your gifts and use them in service to others.

The internal blocks we experience (fears, self-doubt, lack of confidence) show up in our business as self-sabotage (procrastination, perfectionism, playing small.) Sometimes we cannot see these blocks for ourselves; this is called a 'blindspot' and can keep you feeling stuck without knowing why.

One of the biggest blocks I see is overthinking. We are trained as pharmacists to analyze and be logical (for good reason!) However, getting caught in analysis paralysis can leave you feeling frustrated, overwhelmed, and full of fear. Overthinking causes many clients to move into fight/flight/freeze when it comes to taking action or implementing strategies in their business.

How do you shift this? Re-connecting with your heart using a simple Heart Math technique is the easy way to connect to your intuition, which is often turned off because we are so much in the mind. You can have a balance of grounded logic and using your intuition, which allows more flow in your business.

The Heart Math Institute has released over 300 publications helping to establish how heart coherence improves self-regulation and emotional well-being, making it easier to experience peace, positive feelings and a deeper meditative state more quickly.

CONNECT TO YOUR HEART IN 3 STEPS:

#1. Place your hands over your heart, close your eyes, and focus your attention on your heart.

#2. Taking deep, slow breaths, find a smooth easy rhythm of breathing. Breathe in for 5 seconds and exhale for 5 seconds.

#3. Focus on something or someone who you appreciate and care for in your life or simply focus on a feeling of calm and ease. Come back to the room when you feel ready.

As you move throughout your day, you'll be operating more from your heart space and will notice you feel lighter and more at peace.

Reference: "The Science of HeartMath." *HeartMath*, www.heartmath.com/science/.

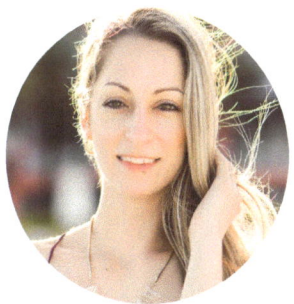

Dr. Christina Fontana is the Founder and CEO of The Pharmacist Coach™ and a Contributing Author for PharmaSis Magazine. Questions and comments regarding this article and further information can be directed to "contact" on www.pharmacistcoach.com.

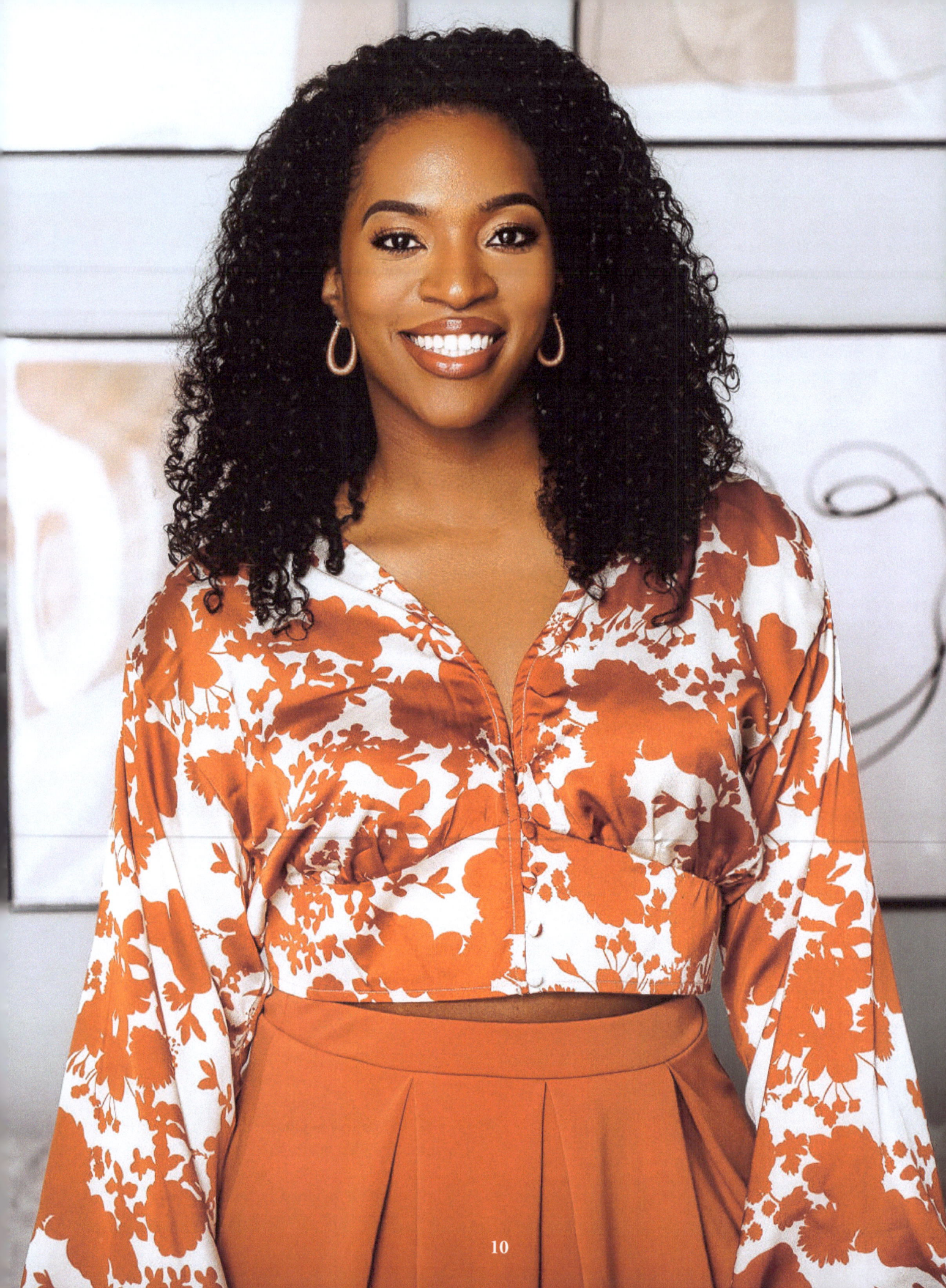

HEALTH WRITING COACH

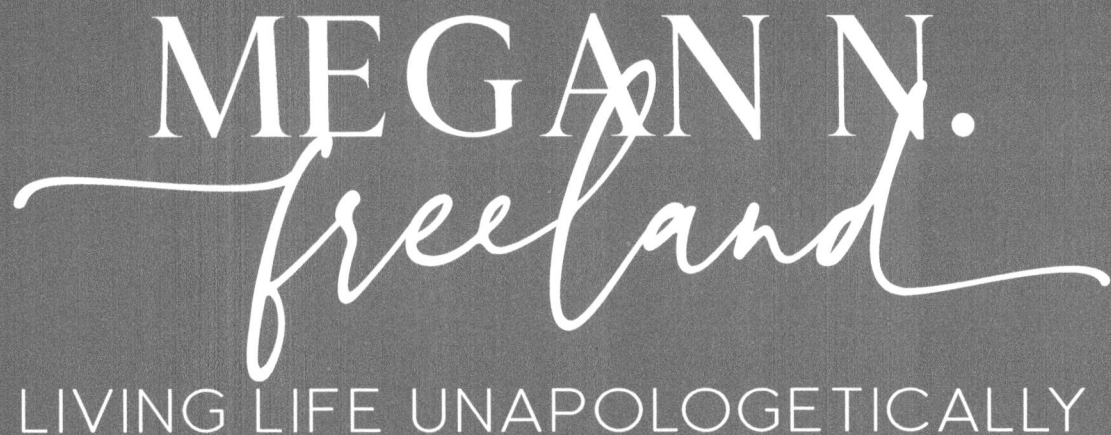

MEGAN N. freeland
LIVING LIFE UNAPOLOGETICALLY

STONE MOUNTAIN, GA | PHARMACY SCHOOL: **MERCER UNIVERSITY** | DEGREES: **BACHELOR OF ARTS, SPANISH; PHARMD,** | PREVIOUS CAREER: **PUBLIC HEALTH PHARMACIST** | NOW CAREER: **HEALTH CONTENT STRATEGIST AND HEALTH WRITING COACH**

Tell your story…how did you get here?

For years, I struggled with shame around never feeling truly settled or content in one space, given my interest in pharmacy *and* public health. Hence, my chosen career path as a "public health pharmacist."

Early on, I identified writing as the skill that could help me bridge my pharmacy education with my passion for public health. I had been writing since my undergraduate years, and I loved it. I even got the opportunity to complete a summer fellowship at the CDC after my second year of pharmacy school. In an ideal world, I would have landed a full-time CDC role right after graduation, but prospects immediately post-grad were thin, so I decided to pursue a pharmaceutical industry fellowship instead.

After a *grueling* yet successful interview and application process, I felt blessed to have multiple offers, but choosing a program was also one of the most difficult decisions.

Nonetheless, I had a choice to make.

The Regulatory Pharmaceutical Fellowship in Drug Information was a 2-year fellowship across 3 different practice sites, including the FDA. At the time, it was one of the few fellowship programs that included a public health experience. Since I couldn't find a job at the CDC, this was the next best available opportunity.

Shortly after the start of my second rotation, the unthinkable happened — *literally* unthinkable, given that I'd had an IUD for about 4 years then. I was pregnant. And I was devastated, to be quite honest.

My career was just getting started and I felt like I had let my mentors down. After all, I was only 6 months into a 2-year program.

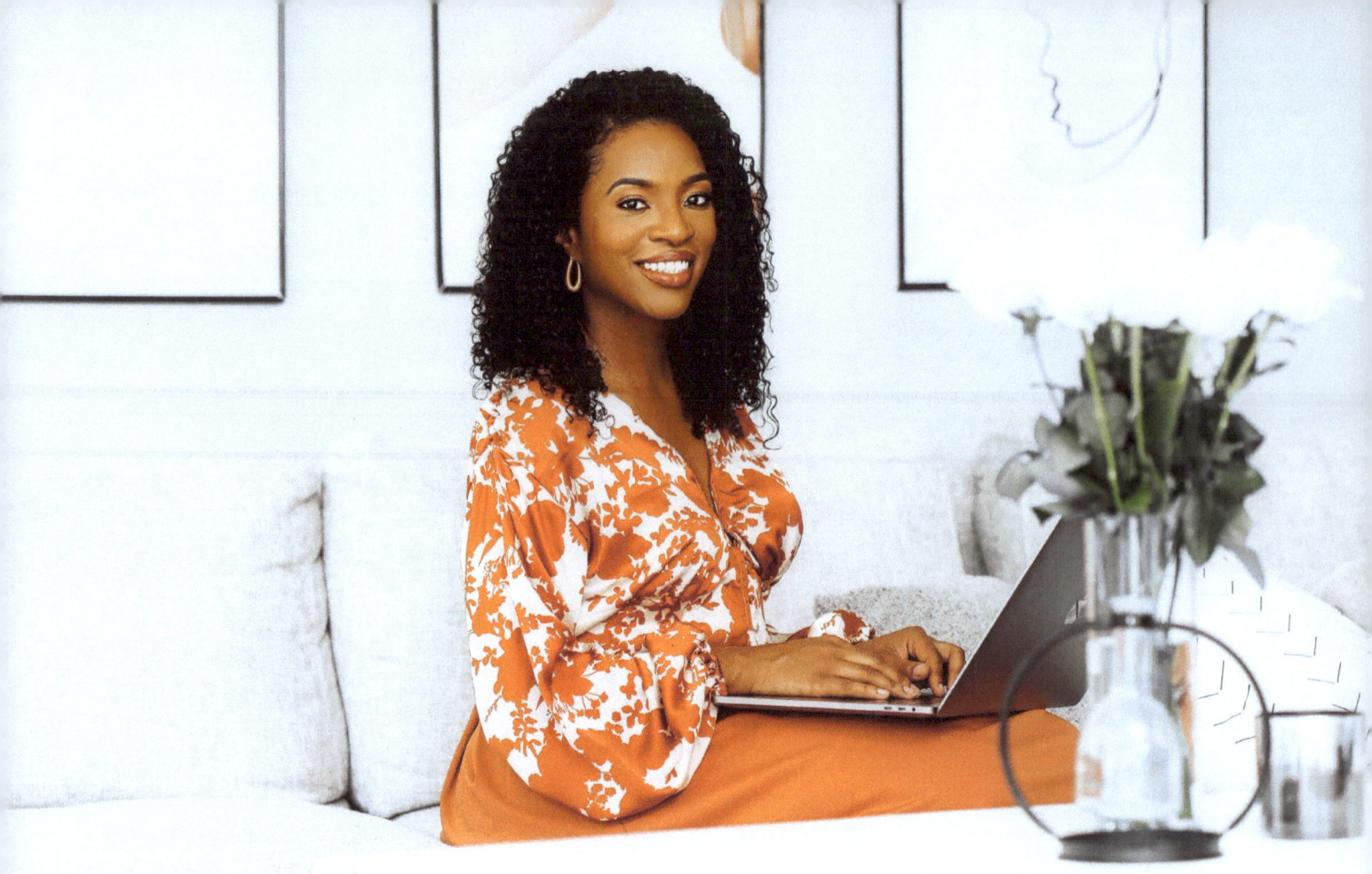

A continuous loop of negative thoughts ran through my mind for weeks. I had "wasted" a coveted fellowship spot because my mentors chose me when they could have chosen someone else. People would see me as "the Black girl who had potential but got pregnant," which would creep into their subconscious minds when evaluating other Black women for the program. I failed because I couldn't see the full program through.

I chose to cut my industry fellowship short by one year to return home in preparation for this unexpected transition into motherhood, which meant that I needed a new J-O-B.

Now, herein lies a lesson on the importance of maintaining your networks. My mentor from the summer CDC fellowship was one of my strongest supporters. While searching for jobs back in Atlanta, I saw that a team within her division was hiring. She introduced me to the hiring manager, and after completing the full application and interview process, I landed a health communications role at the CDC — my dream job!

My post-graduate fellowship mentors used this full-circle moment to emphasize to me that I had not failed, nor had I let anyone down. They explained that the purpose of the fellowship program was to prepare me for a job like the one I had just secured. So in essence, I achieved my goal *and then some* because it didn't even take me a full 2 years to actualize the ultimate intent of the program.

Health comms opened up the world of writing as I knew it. Until that point, I primarily focused on medical writing geared towards health professional audiences. But in this new role, I experienced firsthand the joy of communicating important health information to lay audiences with little-to-no health background.

As my enthusiasm for health communications grew, I began to explore blog writing and developed a deeper understanding and appreciation for health content marketing — the use of health information to engage, educate, and entertain in order to help health companies achieve their business goals. I was **so enamored by the creativity involved in the writing process and the autonomy of being able to generate income for myself that I decided to evolve my side hustle into a full business through StockRose Creative, LLC.**

Describe what you are building/have built.

I've been running StockRose since 2017, with the goal of using health content marketing to fight health misinformation online. Specifically, I help digital health companies create culturally-relevant health content in order to increase brand awareness and improve patient outcomes.

Ever since the beginning of my journey, countless pharmacists — and other health professionals, too — expressed interest in getting to know how I started my health writing business. So this year, it was incredibly exciting to launch the Health Professionals to Health Writers 12-Week Accelerator program that teaches health professionals how to use their clinical expertise to build additional streams of income through health writing.

What's been the biggest surprise about your recent journey?

Taking on a full-time, in-house opportunity has certainly been the biggest and most unexpected development in my journey recently! Aside from that, I think the biggest surprise is that I made it through 2020 in one piece! Digital health saw an unprecedented funding boom in 2020 and work was plentiful, a blessing I don't take for granted at all.

What is/was your biggest fear and how did you face it?

One of my biggest fears in life is mediocrity. So much of my childhood was spent trying *not* to be average. I guess I'm sort of addicted to the feeling of excelling in whatever I do, or at least the process of trying extremely hard to excel.

What is your response to failure?

No one feels good about failing. But setting aside the negative emotions that come along with it, failure can be valuable. Sometimes it teaches us things about ourselves or other people that we wouldn't have learned otherwise. So after the emotional response has passed, my response to failure is to look objectively about what went wrong, what could have gone better, and what I *personally* could have done differently. For me, as long as I've learned something meaningful, it isn't really a failure.

What wisdom have you acquired that you would share with your younger self about your career journey?

Trust yourself. Other people mean well, and their advice is often shared in goodwill, but you're the only person who has to live your life. If I'd have listened to other people, I would be living someone else's life according to their thoughts and values — not my own.

By what leadership principle do you lead yourself and others?

It's not really a formal principle, but the principle I follow is to know myself and try my best to understand others. When you have a grasp on who you are, what you value, and what kind of person (or leader) you aspire to be, it's much easier to trust yourself to make the best moves and decisions you can in any given moment.

But it's not all about you, right? So in addition to becoming intimately in tune with yourself, I find it's also valuable to try to understand the people you work with as well as you possibly can. How do they communicate? How do they manage, delegate, or collaborate? What's their perspective on life? What do they value? What's important to them outside of professional settings?

What would you say to a woman who is unhappy in her current pharmacy role?

First and foremost, "don't let the people get you down!" On a more serious note, one of the downsides of being in a role that makes you unhappy is that unhappiness often seeps out of the work environment and into your personal life. It gets more and more difficult to separate work from home when we're unhappy in either one. My suggestion is to do your best to maintain a sense of joy and peace in your personal life, even if you don't feel it at work. That might require therapy, more time with friends and loved ones, more time alone, or any number of things that help revive your spirit. But without a sense of light somewhere in your life, it will be difficult to find the energy and spark you need in order to move into a better place.

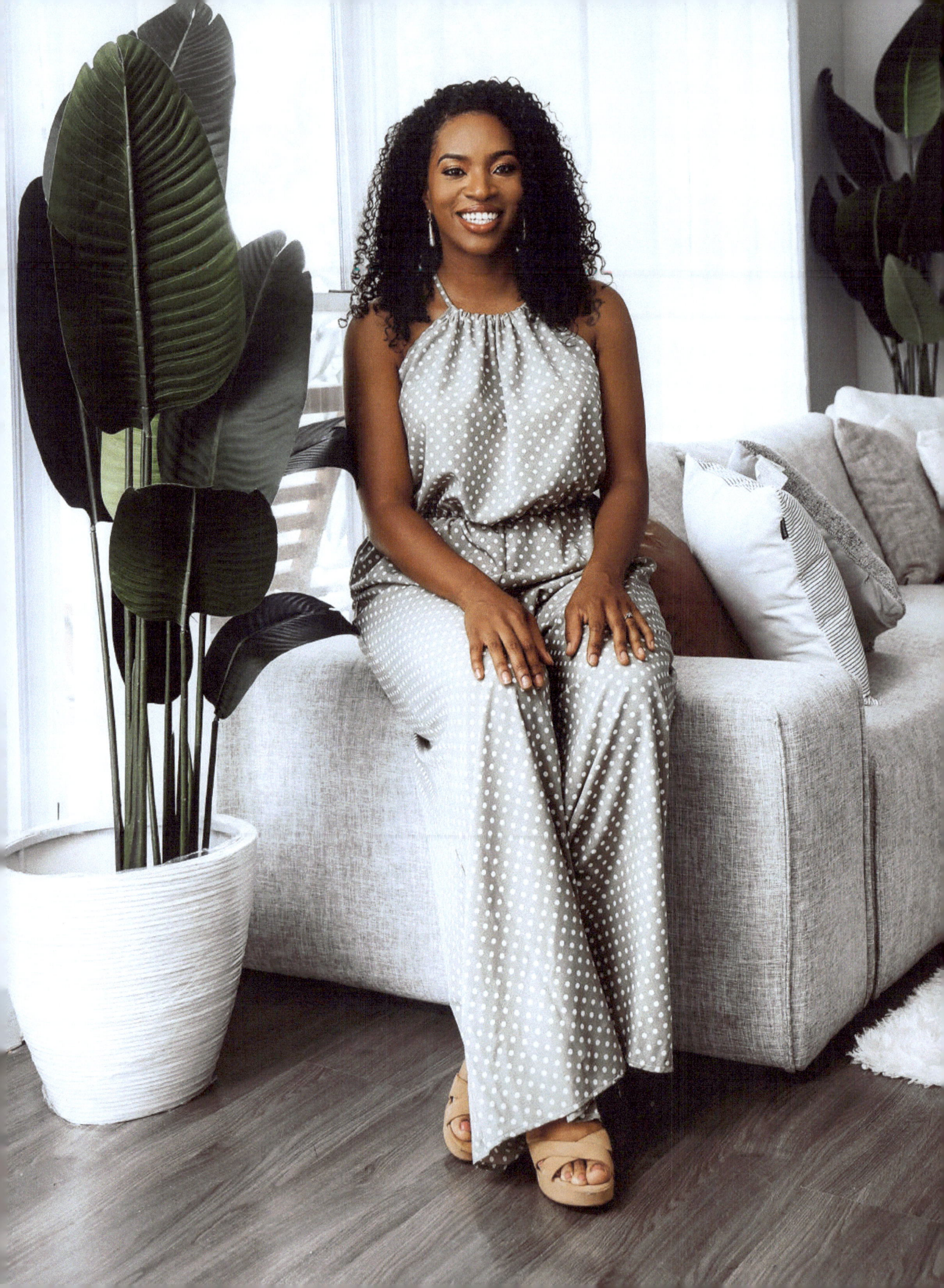

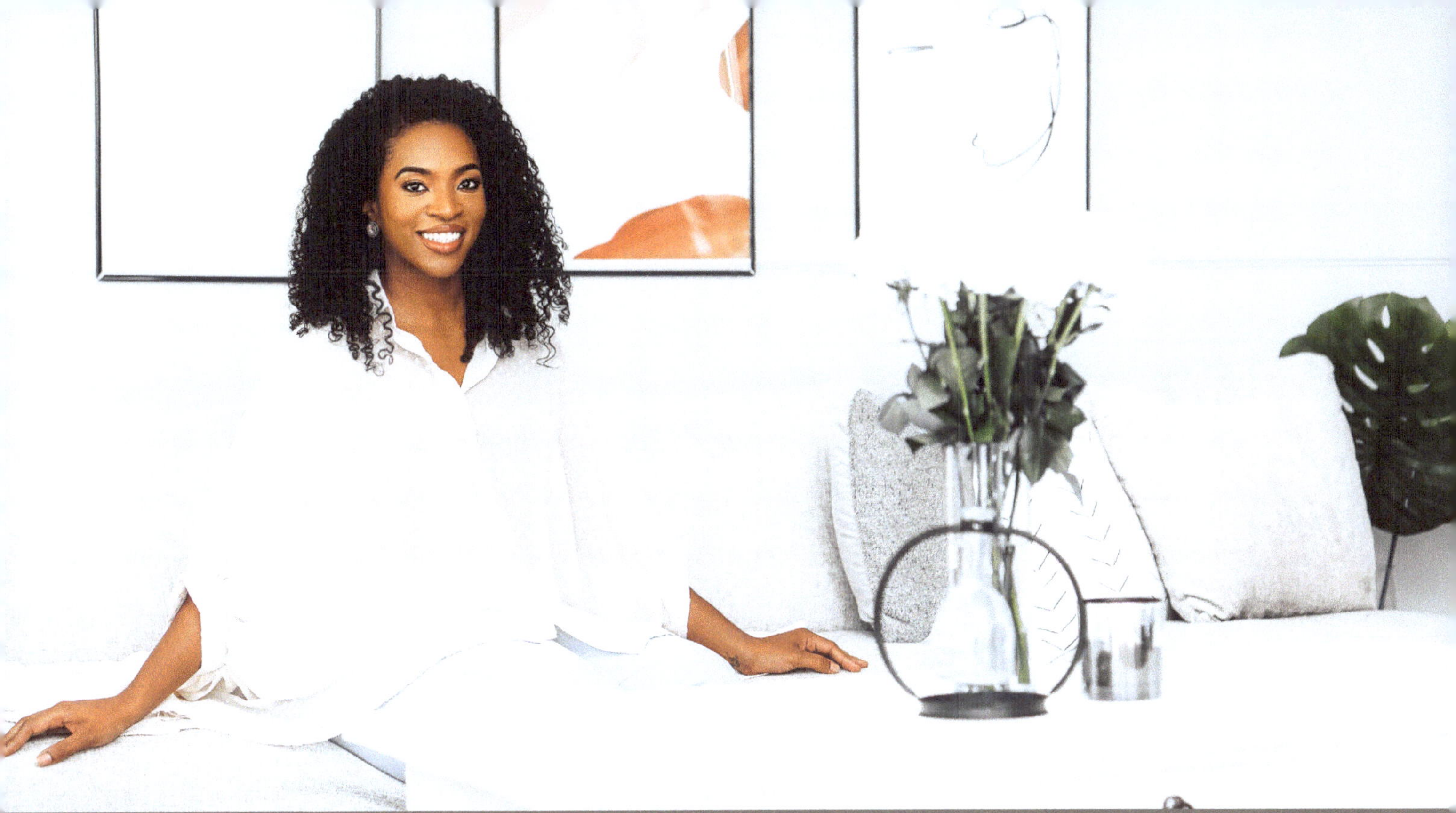

How are you getting back to business in life or business now that we seem to be adjusting to life during the pandemic?

Honestly, I'm just settling into this new, "hybrid" life. My young children are now back in school, and remembering how to work and manage long periods of time has been more tricky than I'd anticipated. I had to train my brain to focus for long chunks of time again because I was so used to having an hour here, thirty minutes there…and piecing it all together. To all the parents out there, cheers to us. We made it!

How do you want to be remembered in your profession?

I would love to be remembered as someone who unapologetically paved her own way and also as a mentor to many. When I say that I paved my own way, I mean that I had the courage to pursue a path that wasn't quite clear with no promise of success. I created that path as I went, but I did so with the help, insight, and support of so many people who wanted to see me succeed. Because of that, it's necessary for me to pay it forward through mentorship.

It's also important to me to represent to *non-pharmacists* the range of skills, talents, and knowledge pharmacists are able to contribute, within and beyond the profession. We owe it to ourselves to show up and show out. Humble season is over. *wink*

What's next for you and/or your business?

I've got to admit — building a burgeoning pipeline of health professionals who are also health writers is one of my favorite accomplishments to date, so I'm extremely excited to continue working with future health writers!

Where can we find you to further connect?

I'm active on LinkedIn. One exciting thing that I started towards the end of 2020 was a weekly video series where I share health writing tips and the behind-the-scenes of what I've been learning on my journey. So feel free to connect with me on LinkedIn to follow along, and let me know if you have any fun names for the series!

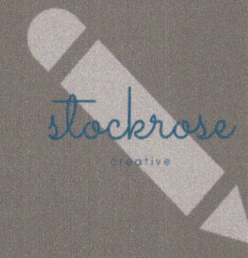

COVER STORY

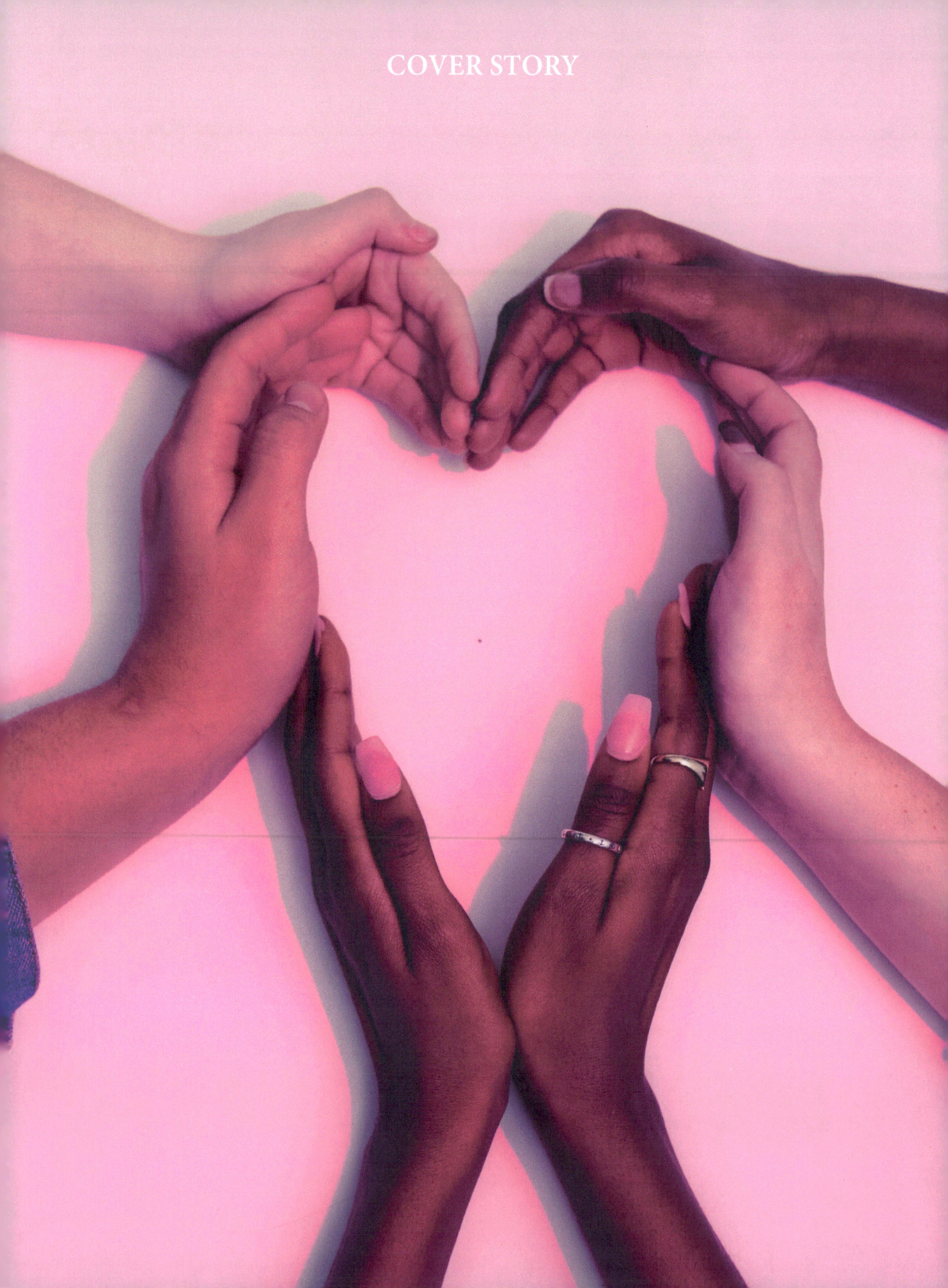

How the 5 Love Languages Could Make Us Better Pharmacists

Written by: Megan N. Freeland

You've probably heard of the five love languages by now. Perhaps you and a partner or friend did the test together. Or maybe you shared your primary love language as an icebreaker on a work Zoom call.

In case you haven't heard of them, the five love languages are pulled from a book called (unsurprisingly) The Five Love Languages: How to Express Heartfelt Commitment to Your Mate. Authored by Gary Chapman, PhD, the book broadly categorizes the way a person shows and receives love into five buckets: Words of Affirmation, Acts of Service, Receiving Gifts, Quality Time, and Physical Touch. The premise is that understanding your love languages and your partner's can help you communicate and love each other better.

Although I was able to predict my own love language before taking the test, I came across a seemingly simple idea in the book that left a lasting impression on me. Chapman explained that we often make the mistake of showing love in the same way we prefer to receive it. But in order for our partners to receive love from us, we must show love to them in their own love languages — not in the love languages *we* prefer.

Mind blown.

It's been years since my partner and I first read the book and completed the quiz, but in recent years I've been thinking about this mistake in the context of non-romantic relationships.

As a public health pharmacist turned health content writer, I'm always striving to communicate health information so that people can understand it, engage with it, and act on it. As a profession, pharmacists of all types must realize that we can't and shouldn't expect our patients and community members to meet us where we are. We have to meet them where *they* are, especially from a communications perspective.

When we provide written information, it should be presented in a way that best fits their individual preferences and values, background, education and health literacy levels, culture, etc. When we're speaking with a patient, we have to do so in a way that the patient can best receive, given their individual preferences and values, background, education and health literacy levels, culture, etc. We should be better at adapting our language and communication styles to the communication styles of the people we have committed to serve.

This doesn't mean that we need to be offensive, infantilizing, or paternalistic. It simply means that we need to be more observant when our patients are communicating to us, identify patterns in their communication styles (e.g., words they use to describe certain conditions, medications, and devices), and apply those patterns to the way we communicate with them. This is how we express our sincere commitment to our patients.

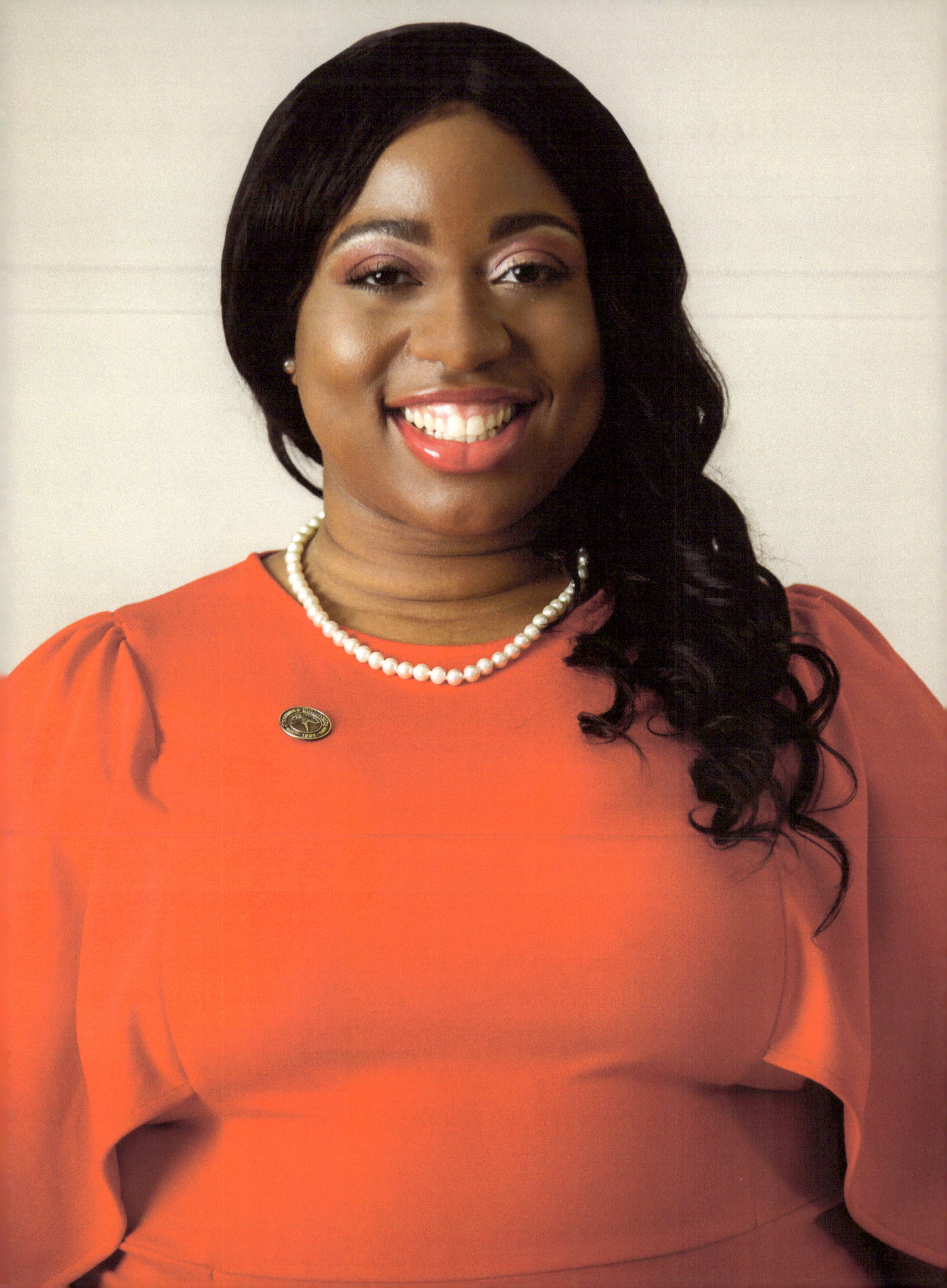

PHARMACY CLAIMS AUDITOR

Keyerrá Michelle Buckley
Showing Up Fearlessly

VINCENNES, IN | PHARMACY SCHOOL: **VINCENNES UNIVERSITY** | DEGREES: **ASSOCIATE OF SCIENCE IN PHARMACY TECHNOLOGY** | CERTIFICATIONS: **CERTIFIED PHARMACY TECHNICIAN THROUGH THE PTCB MEDICATION THERAPY MANAGEMENT CERTIFICATE PROGRAM FOR PHARMACY TECHNICIANS FROM POWERPAK** | PREVIOUS CAREER: **INPATIENT PHARMACY TECHNICIAN PHARMACY SERVICES** | NOW CAREER: **PHARMACY CLAIMS AUDITOR**

Tell your story…how did you get here?

My journey to pharmacy was sudden and unexpected. Initially, I was working for a timeshare company in Florida, but I was unhappy with where my life was at that time. I knew that there was a greater meaning to life, and I wanted to find my true purpose. My mother was diagnosed with Stage 4 Pancreatic Cancer during my senior year in high school and passed three short months later. Being only 18, I did not have much life experience and little support, but I knew I had to make something of myself because I did not have anyone else to depend on. One day, I decided that enough was enough. If I wanted to see a change in my life, I had to be the one to create it. I packed up all I could, sold what I did not need, and moved to Boston. While there, I met a young lady who was currently working as a retail pharmacy technician. She informed me that she completed her pharmacy technician training at JVS Boston, a workforce development organization. Thankfully, after applying and completing the pre-screening exams, I gained entry into the program. I did not have any experience with healthcare other than watching my mother battle her illness, and I was honestly afraid of how that would affect me as a healthcare worker. Once I began my externship and interacting with other

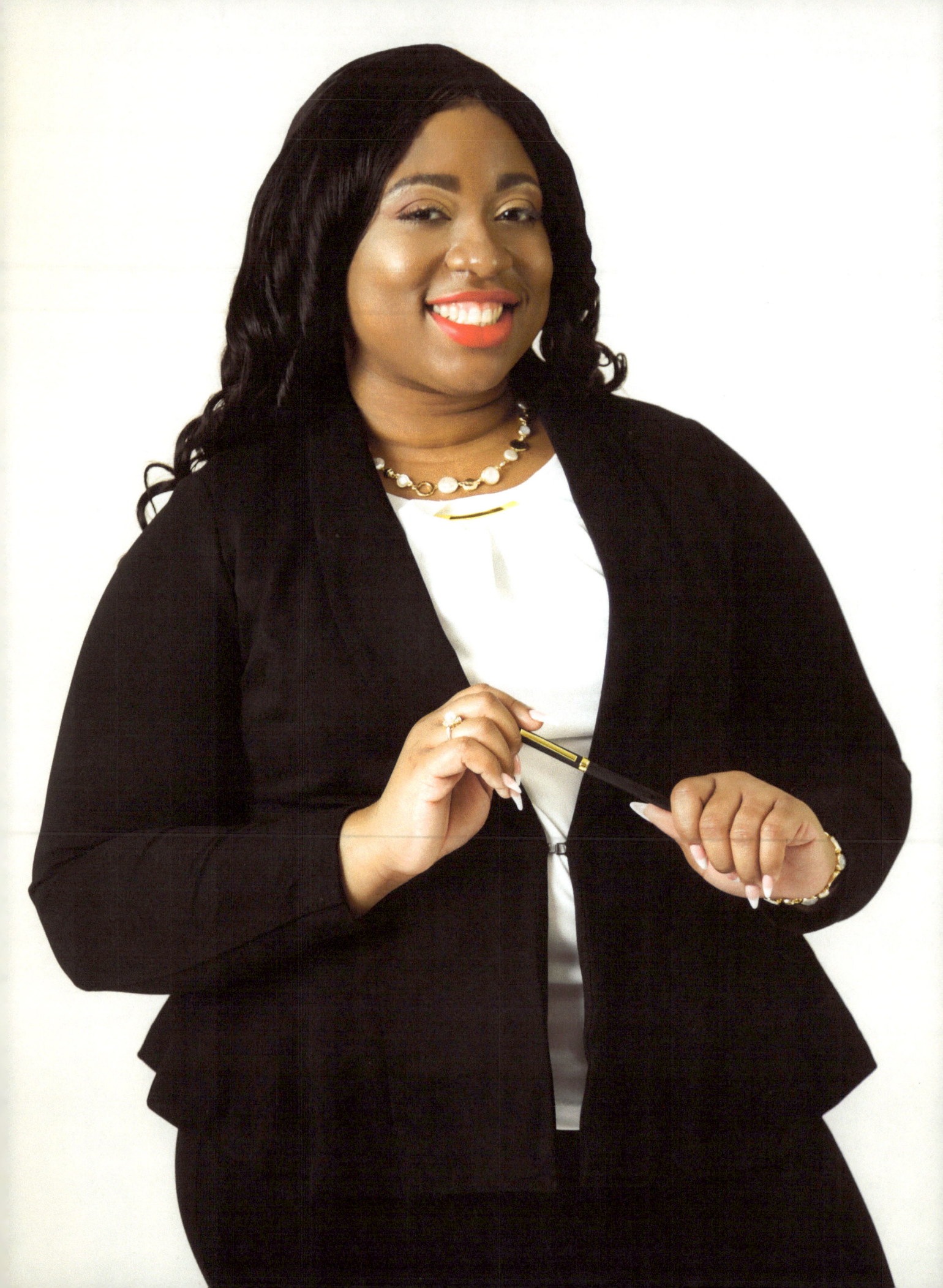

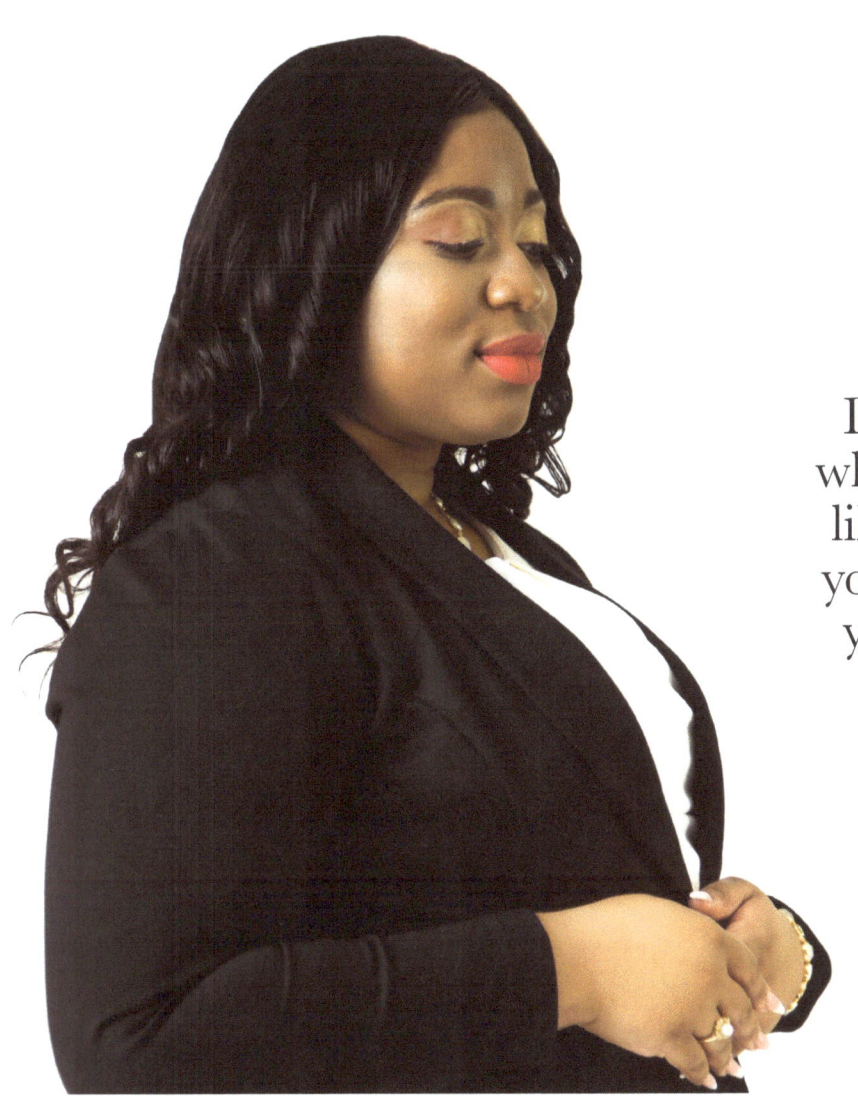

> ## Just show up!
> Despite how you feel, what you think you look like, how much money you have, if you believe you are qualified, just show up!
>
> - Keyerrá

technicians and pharmacists, I knew that despite the difficulties I faced, moving to Boston and enrolling in the Pharmacy Technician Training Program was the best decision I could have ever made for myself. I felt such a great weight lifted off my shoulders as I finally had something stable in my life.

Describe what you are building/have built .

I am currently working as a Pharmacy Claims Auditor and Query Subject Matter Expert (SME) .

As an auditor, I perform comparative analysis of prescription hard copies against processed claim information to determine any errors. Once the investigation is complete, the billing team makes the necessary fee adjustments to account for underpayment, overpayment, and non-compliance fees.

As a query SME, I work with the Data and Analysis team to build queries that detect known and potential billing discrepancies. These queries are also designed around current pharmacy and prescribing laws to ensure state and federal compliance.

Additionally, I am working with the faculty at my university to develop Clinical Research, Health Information Management and Healthcare Informatics education opportunities for students in allied health care degree programs. I strongly advocate for career and technical education opportunities as I am a living witness to how crucial these programs are to those entering the workforce or for those looking to transition to a new career.

What's been the biggest surprise about your recent journey?

The biggest surprise I've recently encountered in my journey is finding my voice again. For so long, I was going through the motions. I was frequently

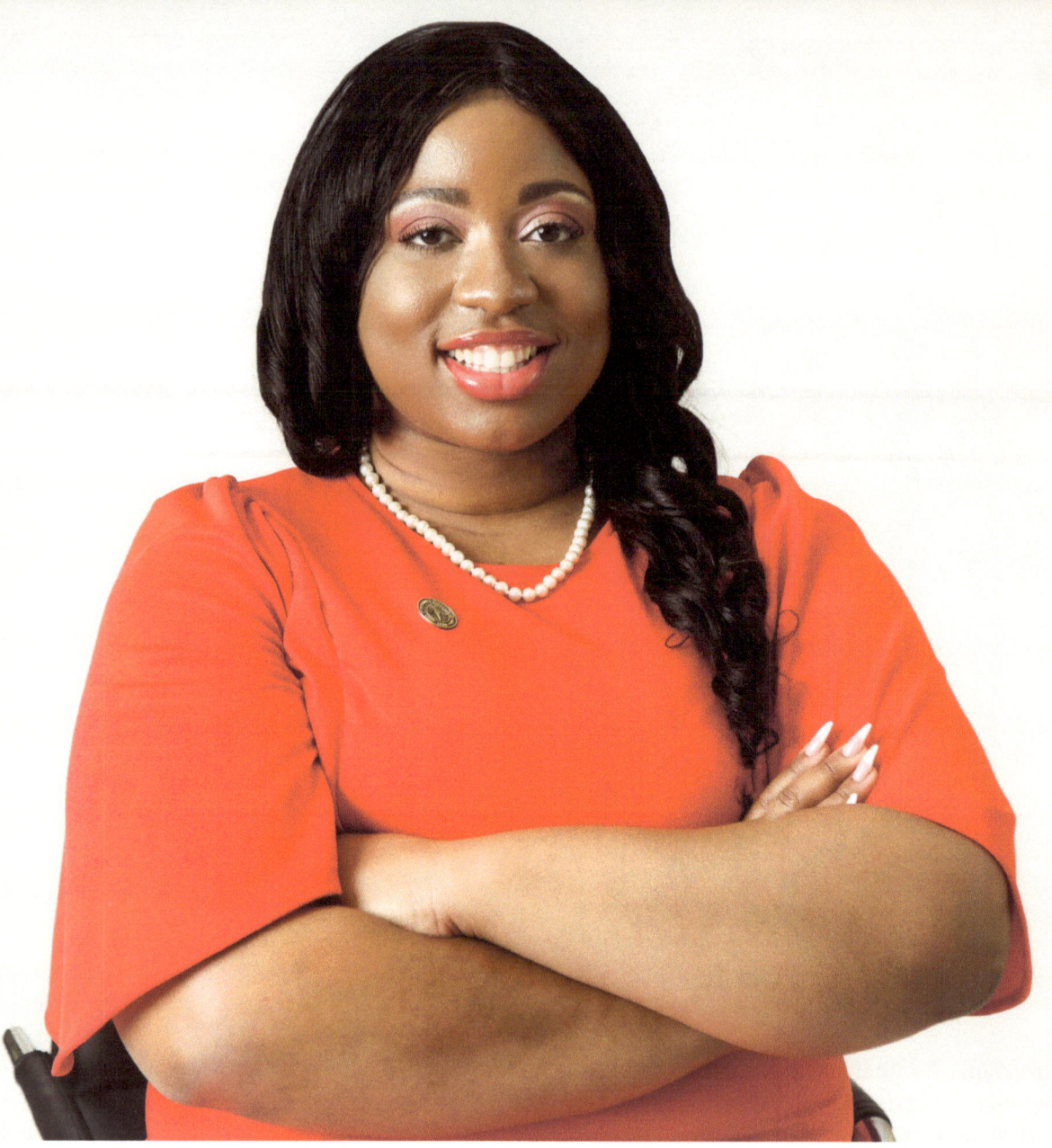

discouraged and reminded of my mistakes until I became silent and numb. In my moments of isolation, I had no other option but to rediscover who I am, who I want to be, and what I must do to get there.

What is/was your biggest fear and how did you face it?

My biggest fear was failure. I was so frozen by my fear of failure that I refused to leave a negative situation that was dreadfully uncomfortable. The pain was familiar, and I preferred to stick with what I knew instead of taking a leap of faith.

After seeking the Lord's guidance, I knew that He wouldn't lead me astray. I finally took a leap of faith to please myself instead of those around me. I packed up for a second time and moved to Indiana to pursue my career and educational goals. I silenced every negative voice and used every ounce of strength I had to create the life I wanted to live. I had to constantly remind myself of my worth, value, and love.

What is your response to failure?

My previous response to failure was to isolate myself. My current response to failure is to dissect and analyze every detail of the situation. I no longer seek success but mastery of my skills. To master my skills, I understood that life will not always give me the outcome I was looking for, but I will always get the outcome I need.

What wisdom have you acquired that you would share with your younger self about your career journey?

First and foremost, I would tell my younger self to leave any situation where I wasn't valued. My time is worth more than any paycheck. Secondly, I would tell my younger self to quickly connect with those in positions I strived to be in. Not necessarily job roles, but with people whose accomplishments lined up with my goals.

By what leadership principle do you lead yourself and others?

Just show up! Despite how you feel, what you think you look like, how much money you have, or if you believe you are qualified, just show up! We miss out on many opportunities due to self-sabotage. Never count yourself out.

What would you say to a woman who is unhappy in her current pharmacy role?

I would tell that woman to go on a deep soul-searching journey. Something special happens when you determine who you are and what you are willing to accept. Once you have figured that out, say no to everything that doesn't fit that image. Secondly, take the time to network with other technicians, join state and national pharmacy organizations, and polish your social media presence. There are various opportunities in pharmacy that you don't even know exist.

How are you getting back to business in life or business now that we seem to adjusting to life during the pandemic?

I am currently strategizing for my next school year. I am in my final year of my bachelor's program, and I have been elected President of the Student Government Association for the 2021-2022 school year. A majority of the students have been off-campus but will be returning in August. I am developing plans and activities to help the students adjust as pain-free as possible and to advocate for them as well.

How do you want to be remembered in your profession?

I want to be remembered as a trailblazer. I want to show new and seasoned technicians the various career pathways they have outside of a retail and hospital setting.

What's next for you and/or your business?

As I wrap up this final school year, I am preparing to take the LSAT and hopefully be admitted into law school next year.

Where can we find you to further connect?

https://www.linkedin.com/in/keyerrabuckley/

TikTok: ms.cpht

FB: https://www.facebook.com/keyerra.buckley

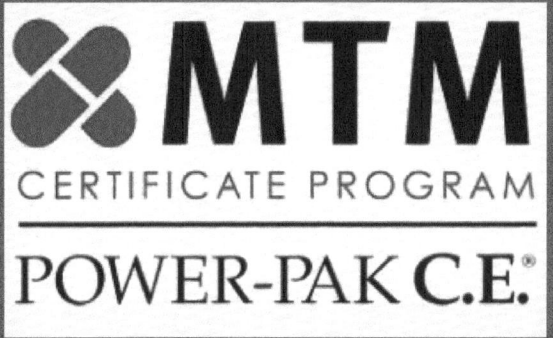

Have you ever thought about STARTING A HEALTH BLOG?

THERE'S A BETTER WAY.

HEALTH PROFESSIONALS TO HEALTH WRITERS

is a 12-week accelerator that teaches health professionals how to use their clinical expertise to build an additional stream of income through health writing.

Starting a blog is a *lot* of work — especially if you aren't that tech savvy.

If blogging has crossed your mind, here are some other thoughts that might have:

You want to get the right health information out to folks...

You think online health information needs to be more understandable and relatable...

You feel that you have more to offer the world than what you can through 1:1 patient interactions...

These are all great reasons to want to write, but starting a blog isn't the best use of your limited time.

There are thousands of existing health companies that already have ready-made audiences listening to what they have to say. If you were a freelance health writer for these companies, they could be listening to you.

Health Professionals to Health Writers helps you begin your freelance health writing journey through:

- **Didactic learning** to teach you the fundamentals of health content writing
- **Experiential practice** to help you build a portfolio
- **Mentorship** to guide you through business essentials like how to find clients and how much to charge

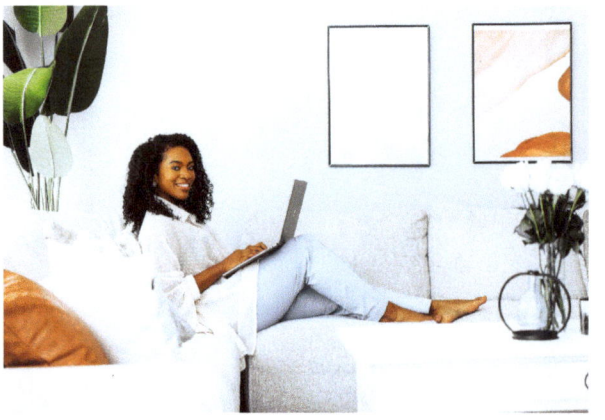

For more info, email
HELLO@MEGANNICHOLE.COM

EVERYTHING IN OUR COUNTRY IS REFUNDABLE BUT FALSE INFORMATION

WRITTEN BY: DR. MANSI SHAH

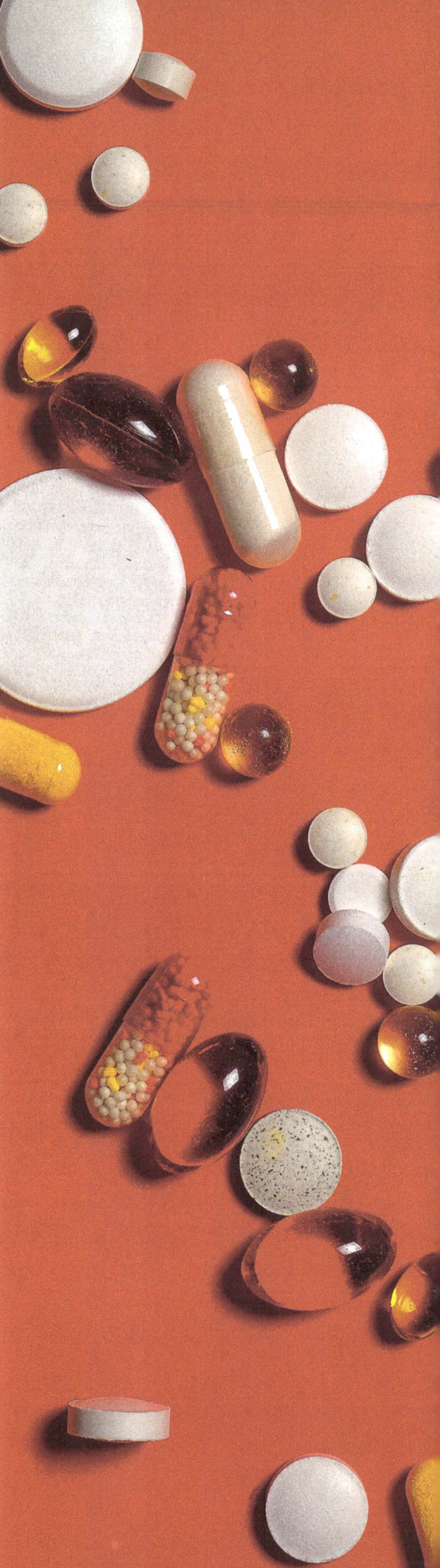

Media, books used in educational systems and studies with apparent clinical significance. I have been evaluating pharmaceutical studies for over a decade and so many red flags are there and rarely I am satisfied with what I see. Actually, at times my biggest question was how this even got approved. Statistically significant drugs are the ones that should be safely approved by FDA but I have seen studies where placebo did better than the actual drug and that drug is still approved.

Did you know pharmaceuticals cannot be advertised in most countries, it's illegal.

Our country is so brainwashed by the big pharma that every other ad if you ever watched TV is about a drug and an amazing visual of this fantastic life that we can live while being on it. I am a pharmacist and I feel it should be banned to show such ads of these medications.

These ads are nothing but a way to emotionally tie people to get their doctors to write these drugs, or if the doctors are prescribing them nobody would really question them.
Medications are not candies or food supplement. Medications should be solely in the hands of doctors and pharmacist, but here it's other way around.

The way we prescribe and dispense drugs here in United States is nothing but a pill mill. Stay alert, do your due diligence. As a nation we suffer because of the deep-rooted problems, I need your support to shed some truth.

Unfortunately, it is all money & power driven and we will be brainwashed to believe on doing things that would benefit the top institutions and that is the truth. Pharmaceutical ads are banned in many countries for the same reason. The Truth is that human race will never have a fair chance to true, honest information ever again. Social media, TV, radio, curriculums everything is leveraged to the institutions benefits.

We are made to believe we are free and in charge but are we really?

The decision to prescribe & manage pharmaceutical drugs should be solely in the hands of healthcare providers without doing any promotions to influence the decision of our naïve patient population.

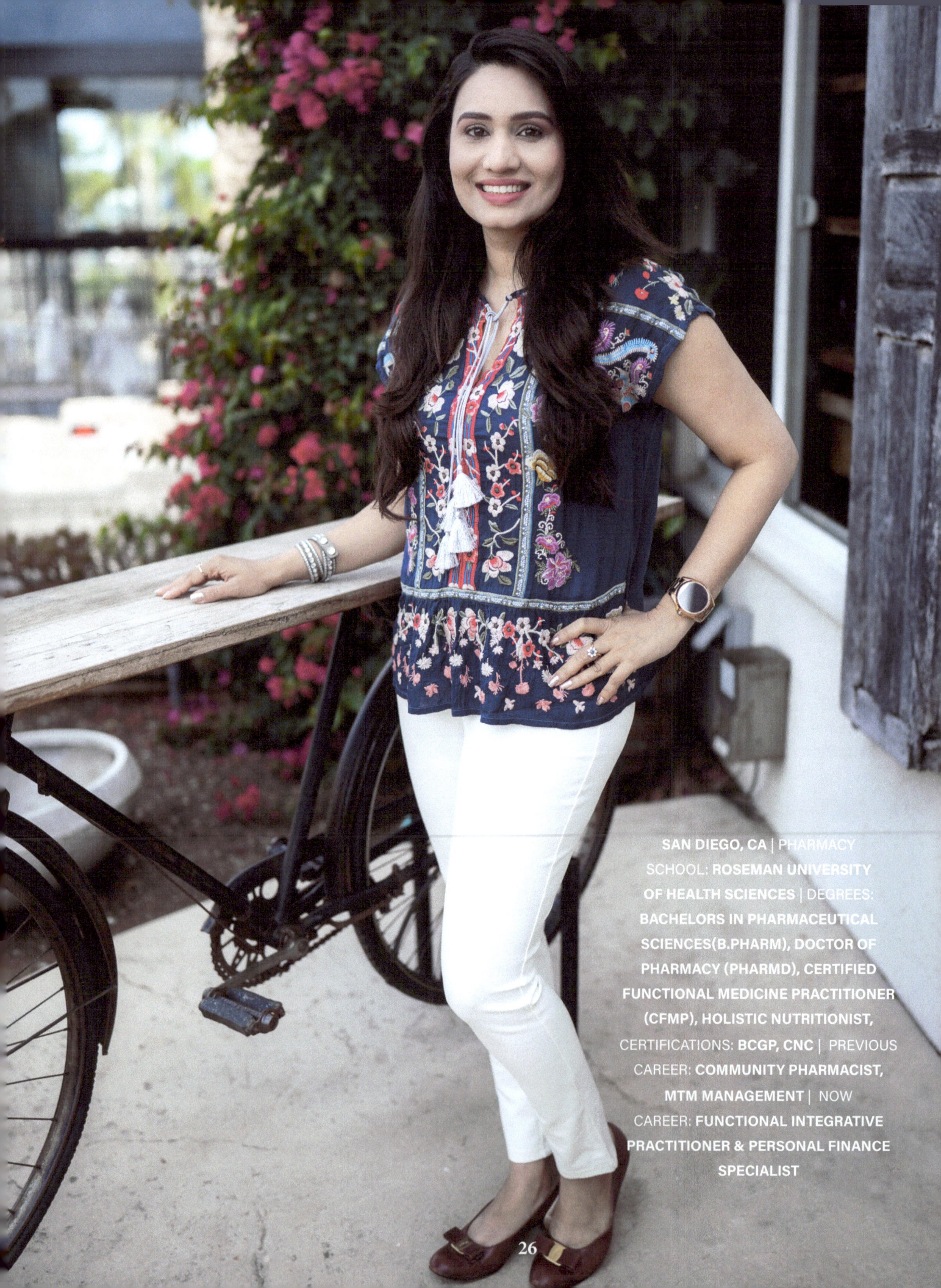

SAN DIEGO, CA | PHARMACY SCHOOL: ROSEMAN UNIVERSITY OF HEALTH SCIENCES | DEGREES: BACHELORS IN PHARMACEUTICAL SCIENCES(B.PHARM), DOCTOR OF PHARMACY (PHARMD), CERTIFIED FUNCTIONAL MEDICINE PRACTITIONER (CFMP), HOLISTIC NUTRITIONIST, CERTIFICATIONS: BCGP, CNC | PREVIOUS CAREER: COMMUNITY PHARMACIST, MTM MANAGEMENT | NOW CAREER: FUNCTIONAL INTEGRATIVE PRACTITIONER & PERSONAL FINANCE SPECIALIST

FUNCTIONAL PHARMACIST

DR. MANSI SHAH

Putting Health Back In Healthcare

Tell your story…how did you get here?

I kept every stone thrown at me because I am building a castle with it.

I am a small-town girl in this big, big world and I am the first generation in my family to be here in united states. I landed Ohare airport when I was just 19 to explore the land of opportunities, my parents are spiritual and vegan, I was lucky to learn a lot of wisdom early on with my grandfather being a yoga instructor in India and Grandma a math teacher and a health enthusiast. So, my journey in wellness and spirituality started young.

It happened that I lost my god father who played a huge role in my upbringing to chronic illness and that is when I decided I wanted to be a clinician to save other people's lives and keep peoples loved ones alive. Not a day goes by without missing him. He is my reason why I am so passionate about helping people with chronic/lifestyle diseases.

I started my undergrad program and got carpel tunnel from stress and then I started my PharmD and got gastric ulcerations from stress and burn out, once again just last year corporate toxicity got me bed ridden. All three times I had to use lifestyle medicine and functional ways of healing, so I started educating myself more and more.

At this point more that I looked around, more evident it was to me that the current system has nothing to do with healing, it is just to keep us marginally alive. Walking down the graduation isle I knew that I wanted to do more in prevention and functional nutrition and lifestyle medicine. I did not see myself surviving in community, hospital, or big pharma. I was able to achieve my dream of building a holistic sanctuary and it was my dream come true with 6th Element- nurturing wellness in 2015 in Baroda, India. I worked extremely hard for it to be successful, but universe wanted something different for me. My toxic divorce took away everything I had built; my ex-husband threw me out of his house one day for being dedicated to 6th element and so I moved back to San Diego to resume a quick fix backup life of being a community pharmacist. I did not mind because I literary had $500 in my account. I started a new chapter in San Diego and was able to build a whole new empire.

I was lucky to have friends who let me crash couches for 3 months till I had enough balance in account and paystubs to show for an apartment of my own. But soon this was going to end I had the feeling as it was never my place to be, after years of dedication and

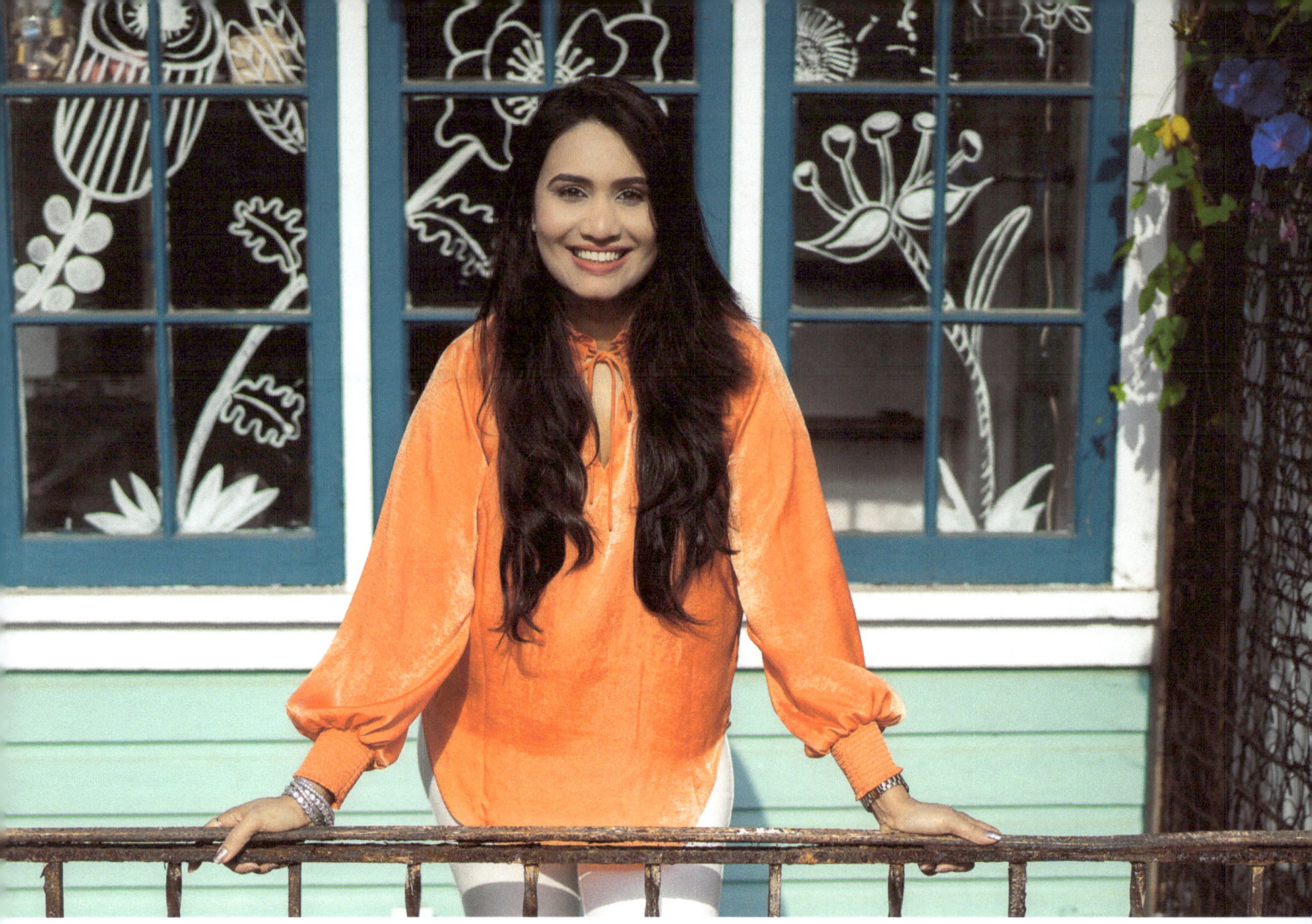

hundreds of great client testimonials one day when another employee complained about me working after clocking out to clean up the store because I literally had no help and was not allowed to put any over time.

I was suddenly violating their policies, hundreds of other managers does the same and I have witnessed it myself. But that does not matter at this point. They decided to let me go in a split second. I had made numerous requests to get more help, many calls and text by my supervisor were never answered.

I did not know how to manage a pharmacy that needs 4 people with just 1 person. I was told by the management that 300 prescriptions a day is slow store and does not need more than one full time technician or an overlap between the pharmacist to cover lunches.

Although just remember that Dreams come true for those who dare to have them. And I had a happy new beginning from this incident of getting terminated.

It was anyways crushing my soul every day to be at a big box that was only focused on pushing unnecessary prescriptions to patients all day. I had patients with over dozen prescriptions and not once I was allowed to talk about managing the medications or help patient with any lifestyle interventions. I felt suffocated and restricted in my life purpose.

So I decided to invest in myself and developed skillsets that can give me a life of freedom and purpose every day that I feel passionate about. Today I have multiple avenues to my career, and I am passionate about helping other pharmacist to lead a fulfilling path with functional medicine and entrepreneurship.

Never again I will feel like I am dreading to work again. I absolutely love what I do now, and it is only the beginning and I invite you to join my talented group at Functional wellness network.

Doors only open for those bold enough to knock hard on them. – Mansi Shah

Describe what you are building/have built (your business)

Functional Wellness Network(FWN) is a dynamic group of like-minded high performing professionals who are committed to putting health back into healthcare.

We are on a mission to building a wholesome functional medicine practice that is sustainable for pharmacist as well as independent pharmacy owners and other modalities of integrative health providers.

What's been the biggest surprise about your recent journey?

It has been so positively mind blowing how many pharmacists are really looking for something different and fulfilling.

What is/was your biggest fear and how did you face it?

The biggest fear was how to replace my corporate income with my business and in the most holistic way where everyone benefits, and it feels satisfying.

I was fortunate to find my mentor Kent Nelson who helped me with his years of mentorship, and we founded Functional wellness network together.

What is your response to failure?

Failure is nothing but one step closer to my goals and grandiose success.

Just like there is no earth without sun and moon, there is no success without failure aka "lessons"

What wisdom have you acquired that you would share with your younger self about your career journey?

If I knew what I know today I would have invested more in my self-development and not in learning how to sell for Big Pharma. I feel I can go tell my younger self, its ok just take a chill, it will all work out in the end. I would ask my younger self to not stress about scores and being the top 5% of the class. Academics is not everything.

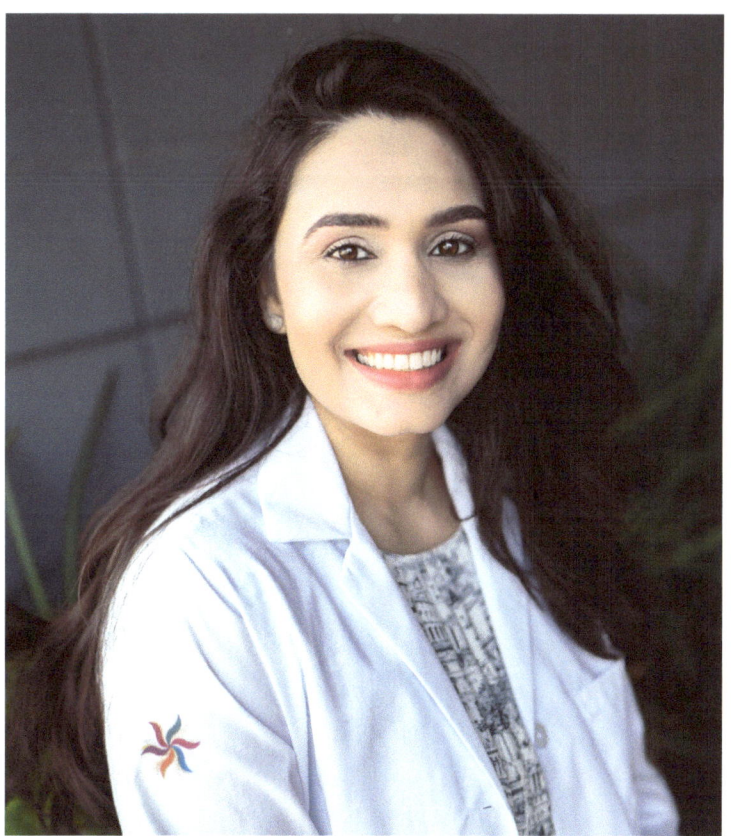

By what leadership principle do you lead yourself and others?

True leaders do not create followers, they create great leader by bringing out the best in other.

A leader is someone who recognizes the talent and potential in others and helps them reach their goals.

I believe it needs a visionary, with commitment and charisma to bring out the best in others, its not about me, its about my team.

What would you say to a woman who is unhappy in her current pharmacy role?

We are not a tree; we can move and we have options.

If you are presented with an amazing opportunity, first say yes and then figure it out how to make it work.

Skepticism and comfort zones kills more dreams than you can ever think.

Just the fact that you are a woman and a pharmacist, you have superpower, and you can achieve great things if you believe in yourself and trust the process.

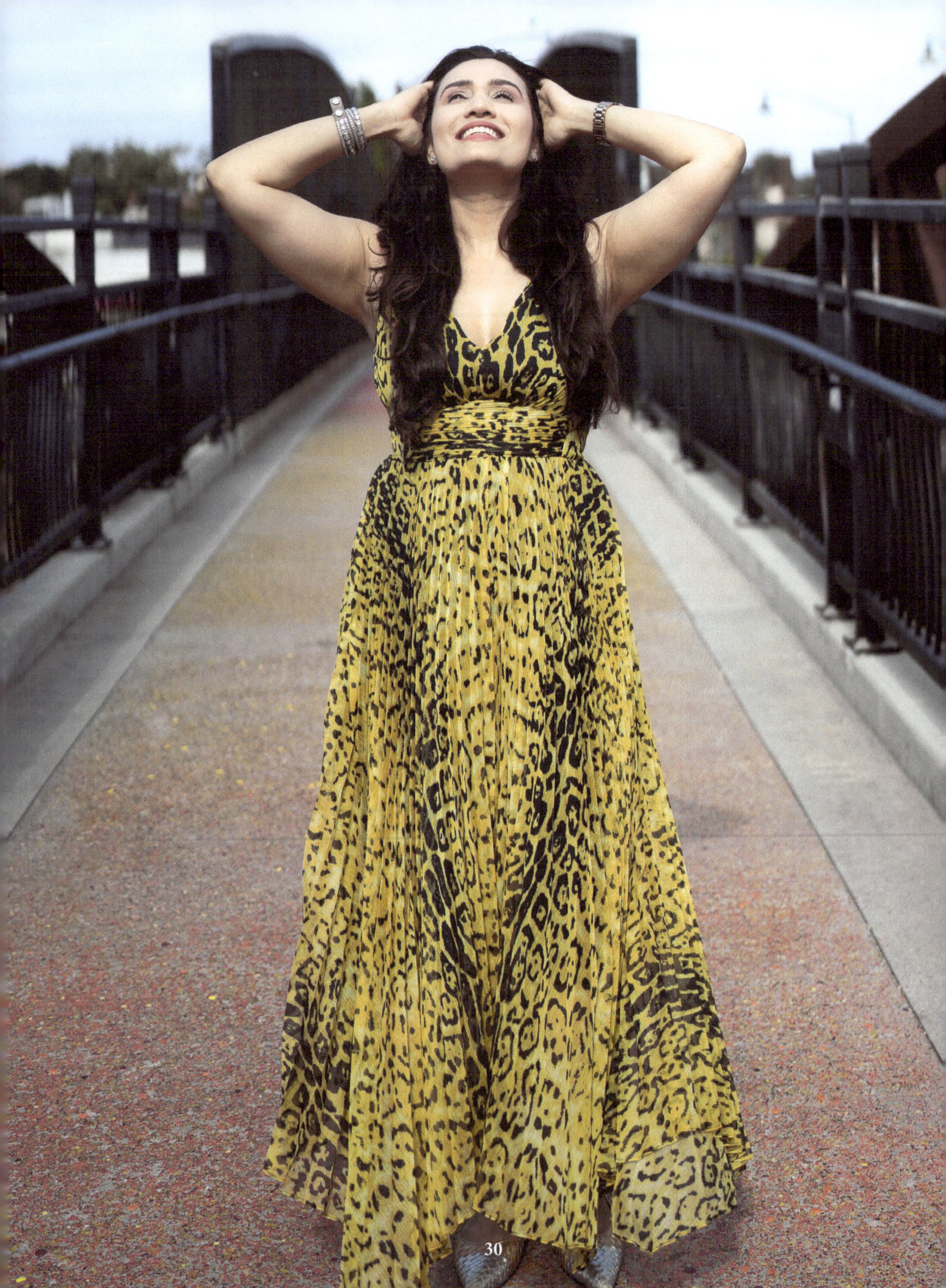

How are you getting back to business in life or business now that we seem to adjusting to life during the pandemic?

Not knowing pandemic was going to happen, I started my business full time in February and with the support of universe I have grown a lot. Now that everything is getting back to being live, I am traveling way more than last year.

How do you want to be remembered in your profession?

I would love to be known as a Functional Pharmacist and a Trend Setter in integrating functional medicine in multiple modalities of healthcare.

What's next for you and/or your business?

Personally, I would like to grow more spiritually and emotionally.

And grow functional wellness network to an exponential level, my goal is to have 35000+ members in their thriving with a new career they never thought could take off just using the skillsets they have.

Where can we find you to further connect?

Functionalwellnessnetwork.com

Join my Thursday webinar or use the contact form, email goes directly to me.

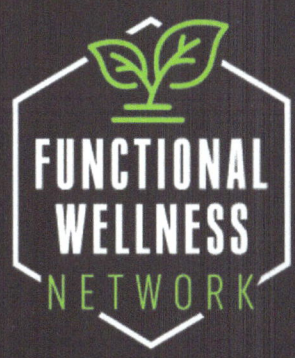

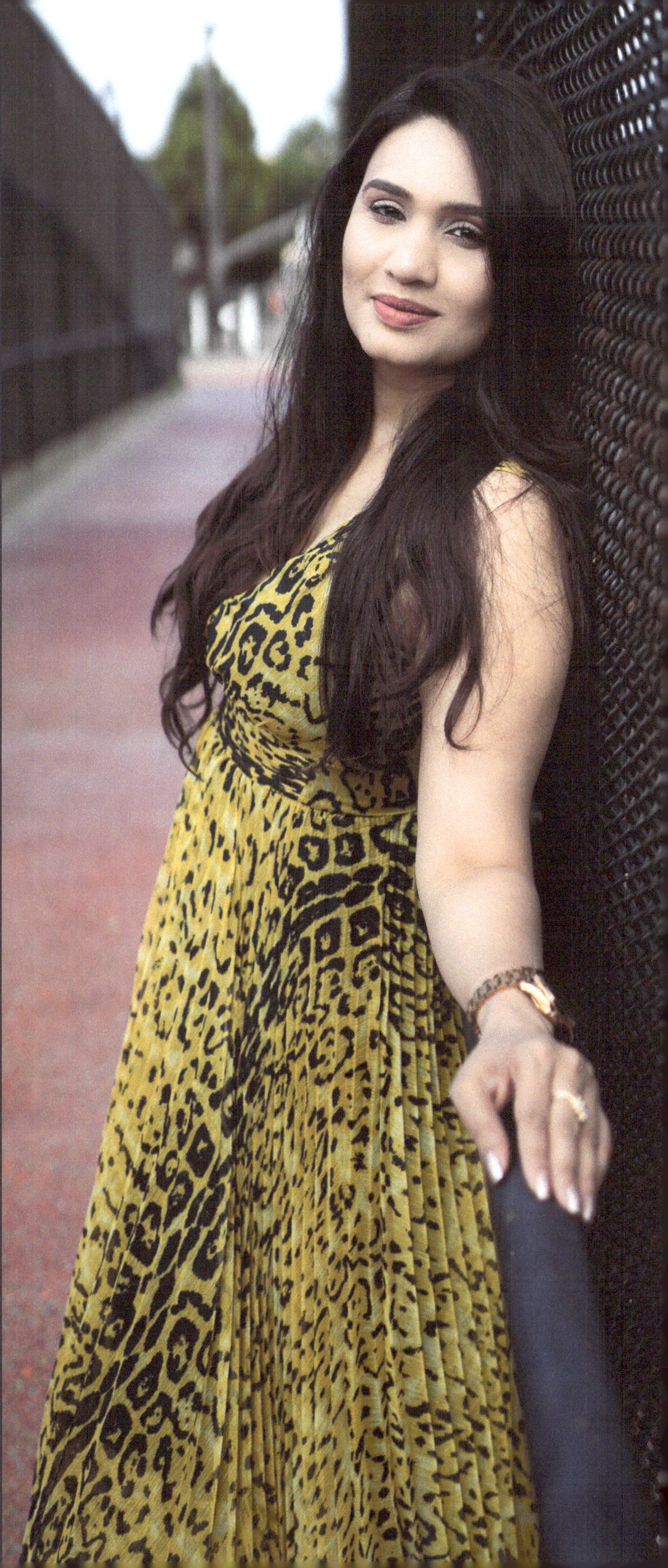

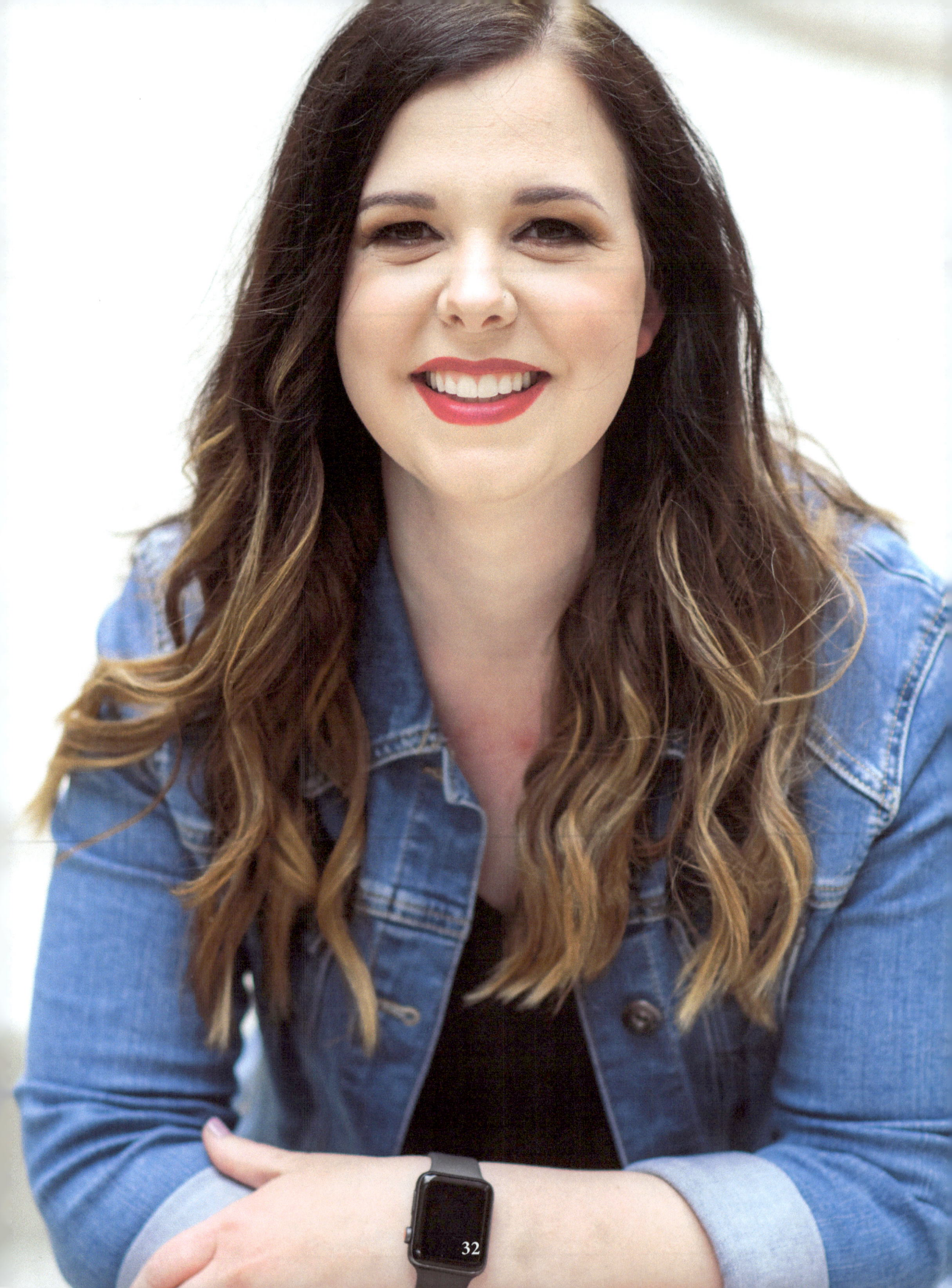

RESILIENCE ENTREPRENEUR

DR. KRISTINE MASON CLINE

THE POWER OF RESILIENCE

Tell your story…how did you get here?

Flash back to an undergraduate college student studying anthropology and working 3 jobs. I woke up at 4am to start waiting tables at a diner in town, followed by night classes, studying while throwing newspapers, then to tending the bar at night. Driving home from work one night I saw a "now hiring" sign outside the pharmacy up the road. Tired of living off of an unpredictable tip-based income, and mostly on a whim, I applied. A few weeks later I found myself turning in waiting tables and throwing newspapers for my first pharmacy job as a technician. I immediately fell in love – I had incredible coworkers that were brilliant and passionate about patient care. I got to see all of the science knowledge I had worked so hard to learn applied to living and breathing human beings right in front of me. So I finished my degree in anthropology and, much to my family's delight, went back to complete the prerequisites for pharmacy school.

Fast-forward after completing pharmacy school (that is a story all by itself!), and I found myself completing a community-based pharmacy administration and leadership residency program. I'm not here to try to fool anyone, residency is hard. There's some analogy here for juggling things that are on fire while riding a unicycle for the first time. In residency you learn so many skills including how to provide and receive feedback, to truly be a lifelong learner, to find joy in work, and how to make the most of limited time. Reflecting on my two years of residency I see how much I grew as a professional and a person. While it was hard work, I loved the opportunity to use my business acumen and analytical approach to support pharmacists and ultimately enhance patient care.

After completing years of post-graduate training, I found myself unemployed. I felt defeated and unqualified. I felt embarrassed to tell colleagues, friends, and family that I was "still looking" when they excitedly asked what I was doing.

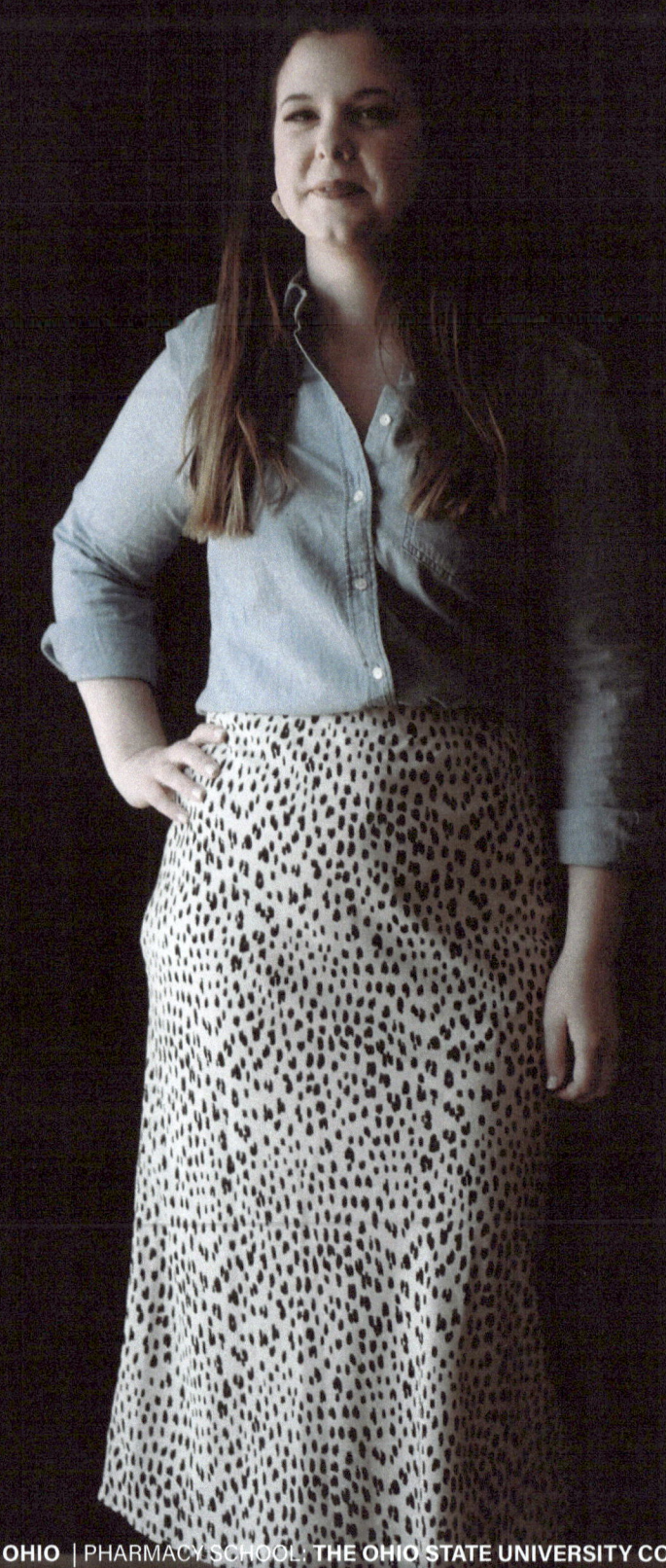

COLUMBUS, OHIO | PHARMACY SCHOOL: **THE OHIO STATE UNIVERSITY COLLEGE OF PHARMACY** | DEGREE: **PHARM D , MASTER OF SCIENCE IN HEALTH-SYSTEM PHARMACY ADMINISTRATION** | TRAINING/CERTIFICATIONS: **ASHP ACCREDITED PGY1/PGY2 RESIDENCY; HEALTH COACH, AMERICAN COUNCIL ON EXERCISE; REGISTERED YOGA TEACHER (RYT-200)** PREVIOUS CAREER: **COMMUNITY PHARMACIST** NOW CAREER: **FACULTY MEMBER & RESILIENCE ENTREPRENEUR**

After months of searching, I decided that I could no longer wait for opportunity to find me, but that I had to go find it. I dove back in and established my own business – where I could apply my skills and expertise outside the four walls of a physical pharmacy. Starting your own business is simultaneously exhilarating and terrifying. I don't know many folks that are excited about submitting paperwork to the secretary of state, but I was giddy with excitement as each step took me closer to my goals.

Once I developed and founded my own business, I felt the world change as I began to live from a place of abundance. People always say that things happen for a reason, and in this moment I truly felt it. Not only did I now have my own business, but I was able to consult on groundbreaking practice changes and began my career as a faculty member.

Each and everyday I make a point to remind myself to fail forward because everything happens for a reason.

Describe what you are building/have built (your business)

I am beyond excited to offer resilience coaching services. You are probably thinking to yourself, what the heck does that mean?? I aim to help clients be the most confident, competent, and efficient versions of themselves to promote holistic well-being and resilience.

Resilience coaching is a very personalized service to either individuals or teams/units. It can include CV review and rebranding, life/health coaching, productivity coaching, or team culture and operations coaching. Ultimately we explore and address what is needed for an individual to become more resilient, or for a team to provide more opportunities for system-wide resilience.

One of my 2020 passion projects was pursuing my yoga teacher certification to be able to offer yoga for individual and team wellness.

What's been the biggest surprise about your recent journey?

I don't know that it is truly a surprise. But along my journey I continue to be amazed and in awe of the incredible women in pharmacy that build each other up, that empower one another, and that work together to make this world a better place.

What is/was your biggest fear and how did you face it?

My biggest fear is fish! But in all seriousness, my biggest fear is not contributing in a meaningful way. It does not matter how many degrees you have earned, how much money you make, or how nice your car is. What matters is the difference you make in the world. I think this fear has been both a blessing and a curse – it has challenged me to try new things, to push myself to be better, and to be present and engaged with others. But it has also caused me to overextend, to say yes *too* often, and ultimately to be burnt out.

What is your response to failure?

I whole heartedly believe that when things don't go as planned, it is part of the bigger journey to learn and grow. It is our opportunity to fail forward.

I hate the word failure. It has so many negative connotations. But that isn't the question, so I'll carry on. After processing the emotions of failure, take a moment to thank it. I know it sounds ridiculous, but each failure in our past has helped us develop into the person and professional we are today.

What wisdom have you acquired that you would share with your younger self about your career journey?

I would tell myself to create boundaries and be comfortable being uncomfortable.

We live in a world juggling competing priorities – entrepreneur, pharmacist, family member, friend (and dog mom). In our culture of workism, where it is not only OK but praised to be always connected and always "on". It takes an incredible amount of practice and self-discipline to create boundaries and stick to them. I can't say that I always get this right, but it is something I am always working on.

By what leadership principle do you lead yourself and others?

TL;DR – Get to know and empower people

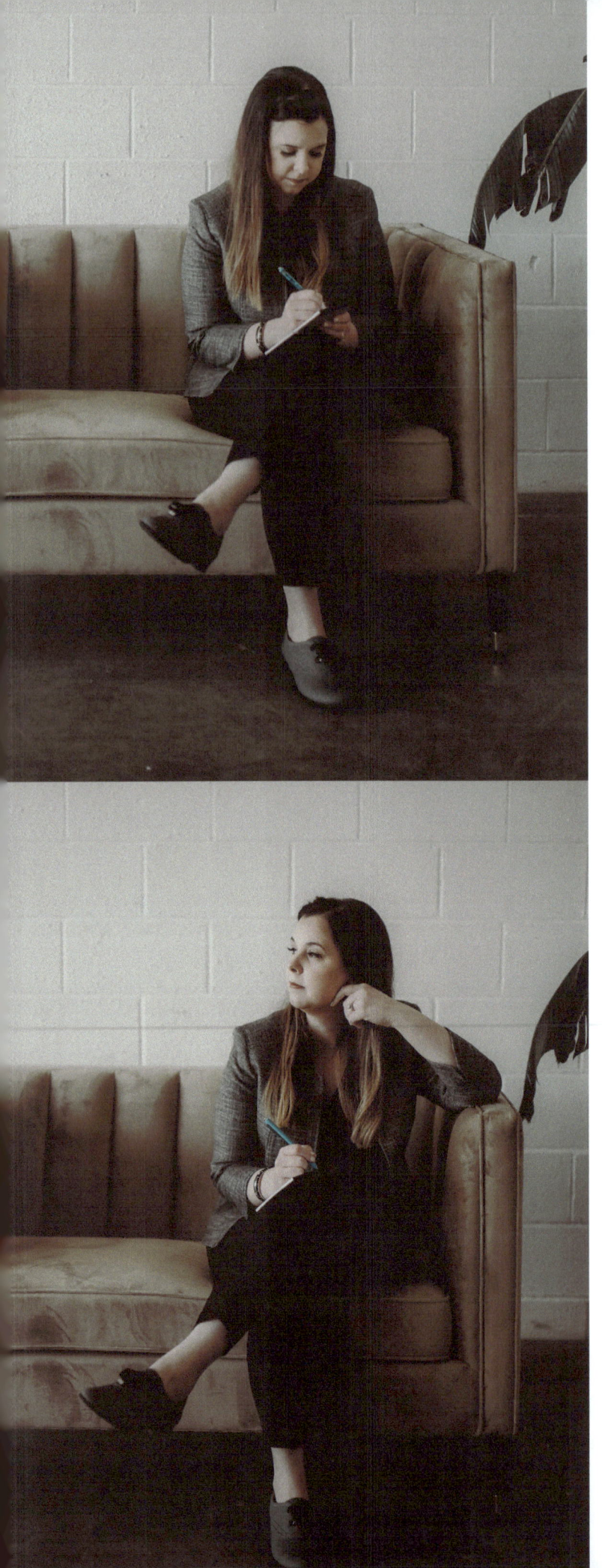

If I look at my results on basically any work-related personality test, I am an outcomes person. Hands down. No questions asked.

Even as someone who is driven and motivated by outcomes, it is vital to understand how to achieve those outcomes/goals. I believe that in order to successfully do that, you have to recognize that *leadership is about people*. When I am in a leadership role (big or little "l" leadership), it is my job to help others be the best versions of themselves and to achieve their goals. Only when all members of the team are included and excelling with the team be successful in achieving their goals.

What would you say to a woman who is unhappy in her current pharmacy role?

Wow, there's a million dollar question. When we are unhappy in our current role it is important to reflect on *why*. It is easy to lean on the annoyances of our day-to-day life, but is that the root? (Let's be honest, we know all roles have pros and cons). Think of stepping back and doing a root-cause analysis on your situation, just keep asking why!

Once we have the root then we can explore - Is there an opportunity to craft your current role into something that you love? If not, how can we leverage current and previous experiences to get to there? Sometimes it is hard to see the forest through the trees, so leverage your support system and resources available to you (like coaches!). I am so grateful to the support I received from mentors, colleagues, friends, and my executive coach.

How are you getting back to business in life or business now that we seem to adjusting to life during the pandemic?

Life during the pandemic was definitely an adjustment for everyone, that's putting it lightly. Our day-to-day lives and ability to care for ourselves as a whole person changed. I took the opportunity to look for other "tools in the toolkit" during my time at home, including becoming a registered yoga teacher.

I am very grateful that I have been able to connect

with more folks than ever before in our virtual world, through conferences, webinars, and social media. The comfort with virtual/tele-connections is one of the silver linings of 2020.

But I am *beyond* excited to start to work with clients and attend speaking engagements in-person again!

How do you want to be remembered in your profession?

One phrase that sits with me is that you aren't remembered for what you say, or what you do; but you are remembered for how you make people feel.

I don't believe that I as an individual need to be remembered, but I do hope that I can help others remember the feelings of empowerment and motivation – that I help them to be reminded of the badass women they are, and my hope is that they pay it forward.

What's next for you and/or your business?

I am excited to continue working with individuals and teams to set them up for successful and sustainable resilience, and to collaborate with folks through speaking engagements. It is truly an honor to connect with so many beautiful souls across the country.

Where can we find you to further connect?

Instagram: @drkristinecline

Website: drkristinecline.com

RESILIENT REBRAND	BUILD RESILIENCE	FOSTER RESILIENCE
CV & BRAND COACHING	PERSONAL COACHING	TEAM COACHING

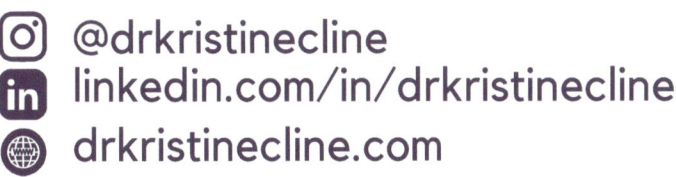

@drkristinecline
linkedin.com/in/drkristinecline
drkristinecline.com

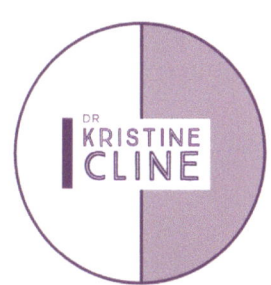

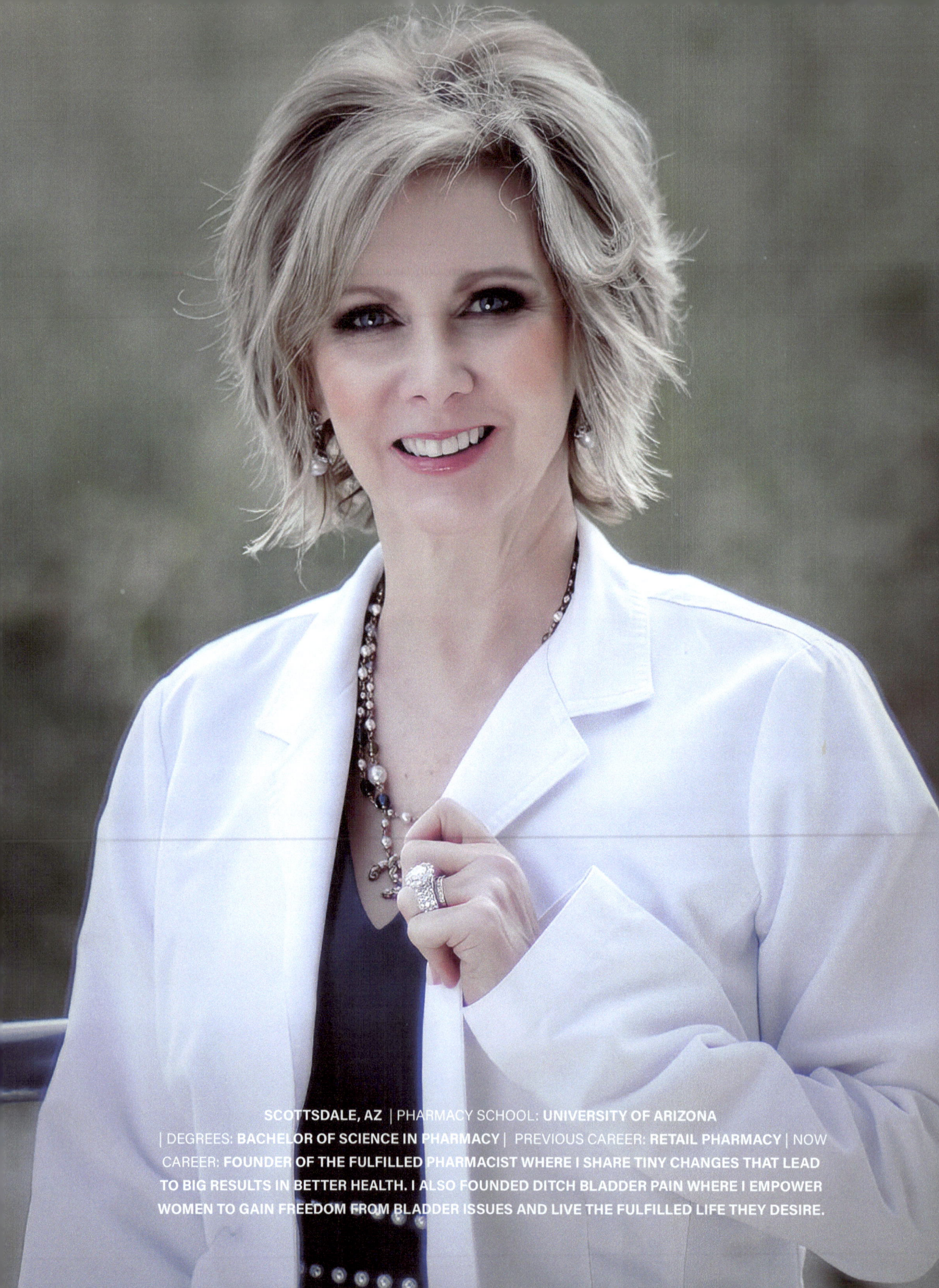

SCOTTSDALE, AZ | PHARMACY SCHOOL: **UNIVERSITY OF ARIZONA** | DEGREES: **BACHELOR OF SCIENCE IN PHARMACY** | PREVIOUS CAREER: **RETAIL PHARMACY** | NOW CAREER: **FOUNDER OF THE FULFILLED PHARMACIST WHERE I SHARE TINY CHANGES THAT LEAD TO BIG RESULTS IN BETTER HEALTH. I ALSO FOUNDED DITCH BLADDER PAIN WHERE I EMPOWER WOMEN TO GAIN FREEDOM FROM BLADDER ISSUES AND LIVE THE FULFILLED LIFE THEY DESIRE.**

SOCIAL PHARMACIST

LISA KING, RPH

The Fulfilled Pharmacist

Tell your story…how did you get here?

I have always been passionate about sharing health and wellness whether inside or outside of the pharmacy. I love being a pharmacist and have enjoyed a long career in this wonderful profession. I was lucky enough to marry my high school sweetheart and we have a growing family.

Despite all of my blessings, I felt I wanted more. I wanted more fulfillment, more satisfaction, more knowing I was making a difference in the lives of others. I have always been proud of being a pharmacist and felt it was a career choice that could touch many lives. However, I found myself at a point where I felt frustrated that I could not find my true purpose. Eventually through a series of unexpected twists and turns, I started sharing about bladder health. This has brought me just what I was looking for in my journey to find more. I know now my more is to bring hope to women experiencing bladder issues.

Bladder issues are surrounded by stigma and embarrassment. This was definitely not a topic I thought I would ever be sharing! I was diagnosed with Interstitial Cystitis (Painful Bladder Syndrome) twenty -seven years ago. This is an extremely painful diagnosis, yet I never gave up hope. I expected that one day I that would be able to live my life the way that I wanted to without the worry, shame and guilt that surrounds bladder issues.

When I coauthored the book *Tiny Life Changes* with my sister, I was invited to be a guest on many midlife podcasts. During one podcast the conversation turned to my painful bladder diagnoses. I soon thought "Oh no!" "Why?" This was something I really did not want to put into my present as I was so grateful to have moved past this difficult diagnosis.

After answering this question on this podcast, I was soon asked about this topic again and again as I had also previously mentioned it on social media once as well. Suddenly, I was getting messages from women who were suffering in silence with bladder issues.

I knew I had to put my own reservations aside on sharing about this sensitive subject matter and I needed to share my story! My hope in sharing my story is always to give hope to women who may have bladder issues. Many women feel extremely alone in this journey and my intent is always to let them know they are not alone and there are treatment options!

Now through my website www.ditchbladderpain.com and through media and social media I am giving a voice to those women.

Describe what you are building/have built (your business)

Through my website and my social media platforms, I am bringing an awareness to bladder issues. This is something that is often not discussed due to the shame and stigma that can surround this issue. I have collaborated with drug manufacturers, other health care professionals and even shared on Oprah.com on issues surrounding overactive and painful bladder.

What's been the biggest surprise about your recent journey?

What has surprised me most about the journey is how much I truly feel like a pharmacist when sharing on this subject. Whether it be Overactive Bladder, Painful Bladder or Recurrent Urinary Tract Infections; bladder issues often aren't discussed. I love supporting and encouraging the women who reach out to me. I have also been very surprised as to how many women reach out to me to share on their own platforms as well. There have been so many wonderful women supporting me in sharing this message. I have truly experienced women supporting women through the women I have met on social media!

What is/was your biggest fear and how did you face it?

At times this subject can be embarrassing to discuss even for me! I was extremely shy as a child and now I am advocating on a very embarrassing subject. I move past these feelings and fears and know this is my purpose in life. I am here to empower women to gain freedom from bladder issues!

What is your response to failure?

I am extremely resilient. My favorite quote is "Fall down seven times, get up eight". I truly do not look at any situation as a failure but more as a learning lesson. What can I do differently to have a different outcome? I also love to say YES before I say NO. I stay open to possibilities and that is how I wound up where I am today. I went from sharing about general health and wellness to coauthoring a book which then lead to me sharing about bladder health! When I first started sharing on social media, I would never have imagined that I would be where I am today; a voice for women who have bladder issues!

What wisdom have you acquired that you would share with your younger self about your career journey?

The advice I would share with myself is to keep shining my light! When I coauthored "Tiny Life Changes" with my sister, I made a vow to myself. My vow was to not hide my light under a bushel. I knew we had an important message and I wanted to share it everywhere. There were days others questioned my presence on social media. I still hold this thought today. When you shine your light, it does two things. It allows others to shine their light along with you. It also lights a path for others who may be living in darkness. When giving hope to women living with bladder issues, my desire is to reach just one. If I shine a light on a dark path for even one woman who may be living in fear and frustration, I know that I have achieved my goal. I always aspire to shine that light and give that hope!

By what leadership principle do you lead yourself and others?

I lead by example through mentoring others and always look towards the positive. For many years of my career I was a preceptor to pharmacy students. I enjoy working with pharmacy students because they bring such vibrancy to the profession. I love sharing my love for pharmacy especially through patient care. As a retail pharmacist, I know I have touched many lives and they have touched mine as well! Getting to know patients on an intimate level has been the most gratifying part of my career

What would you say to a woman who is unhappy in her current pharmacy role?

There are career options and you can experience joy and fulfillment as a pharmacist; take it one step and one day at a time! As a pharmacist of 33 years, I have seen the profession change considerably during my career. Many pharmacists can feel extremely overwhelmed and unfulfilled due to current work conditions. If it is not a possibility to leave the current work situation, do one thing daily that will get you closer to your goal. Start networking with others, register the name of the company you want to start, research career options. Just start! Doing even small things daily will move you forward towards the changes that you want to make in your life and career. Keep going, you will soon reach your goal!

How are you getting back to business in life or business now that we seem to adjusting to life during the pandemic?

The pandemic has taught me to SLOW down! I am working on being present in the lives of my family and being content to just be. For many years, as with most pharmacists, I was doing, doing, doing. There was always a feeling that I was not doing enough whether that was originally studying in school, performing at

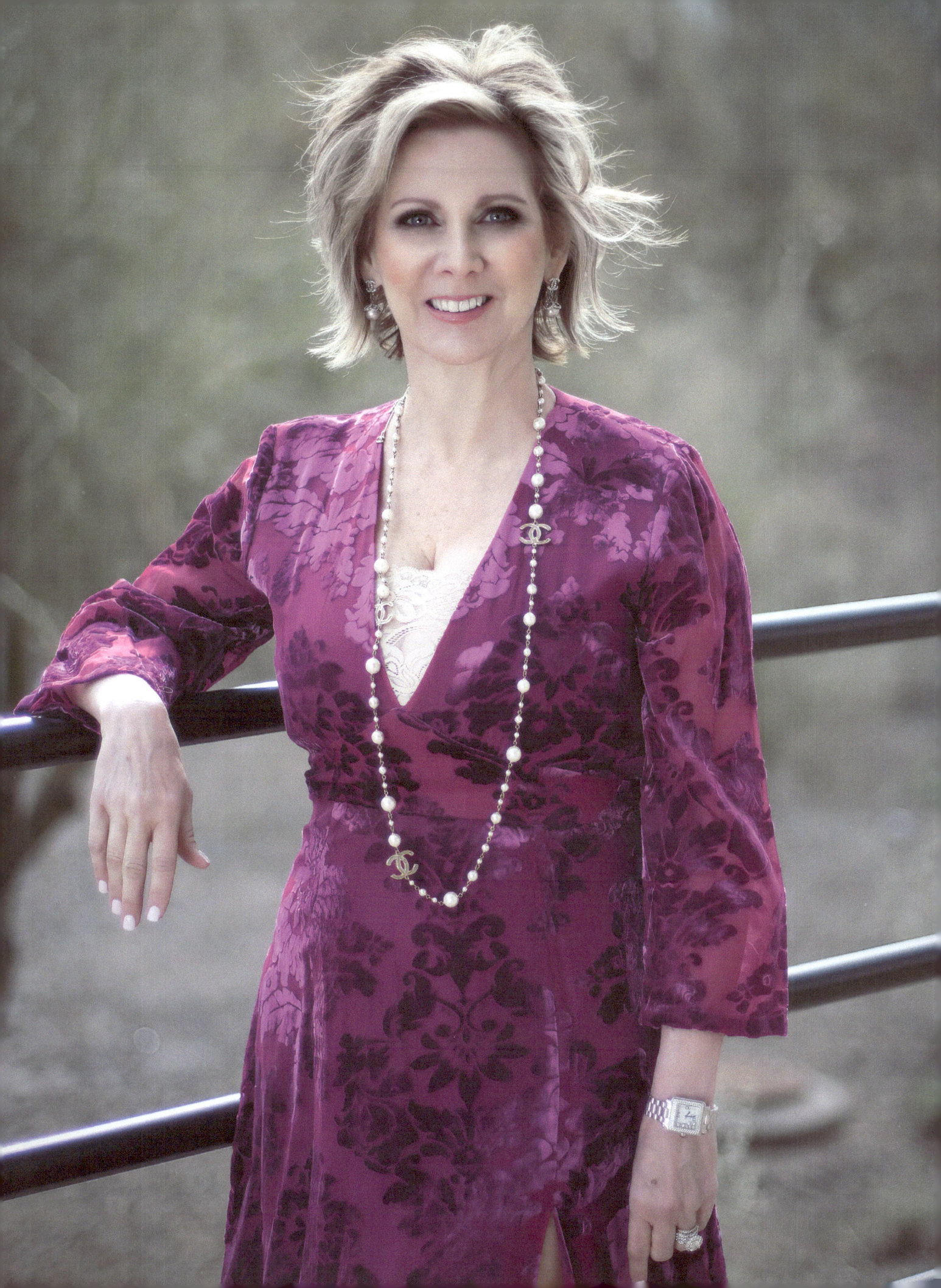

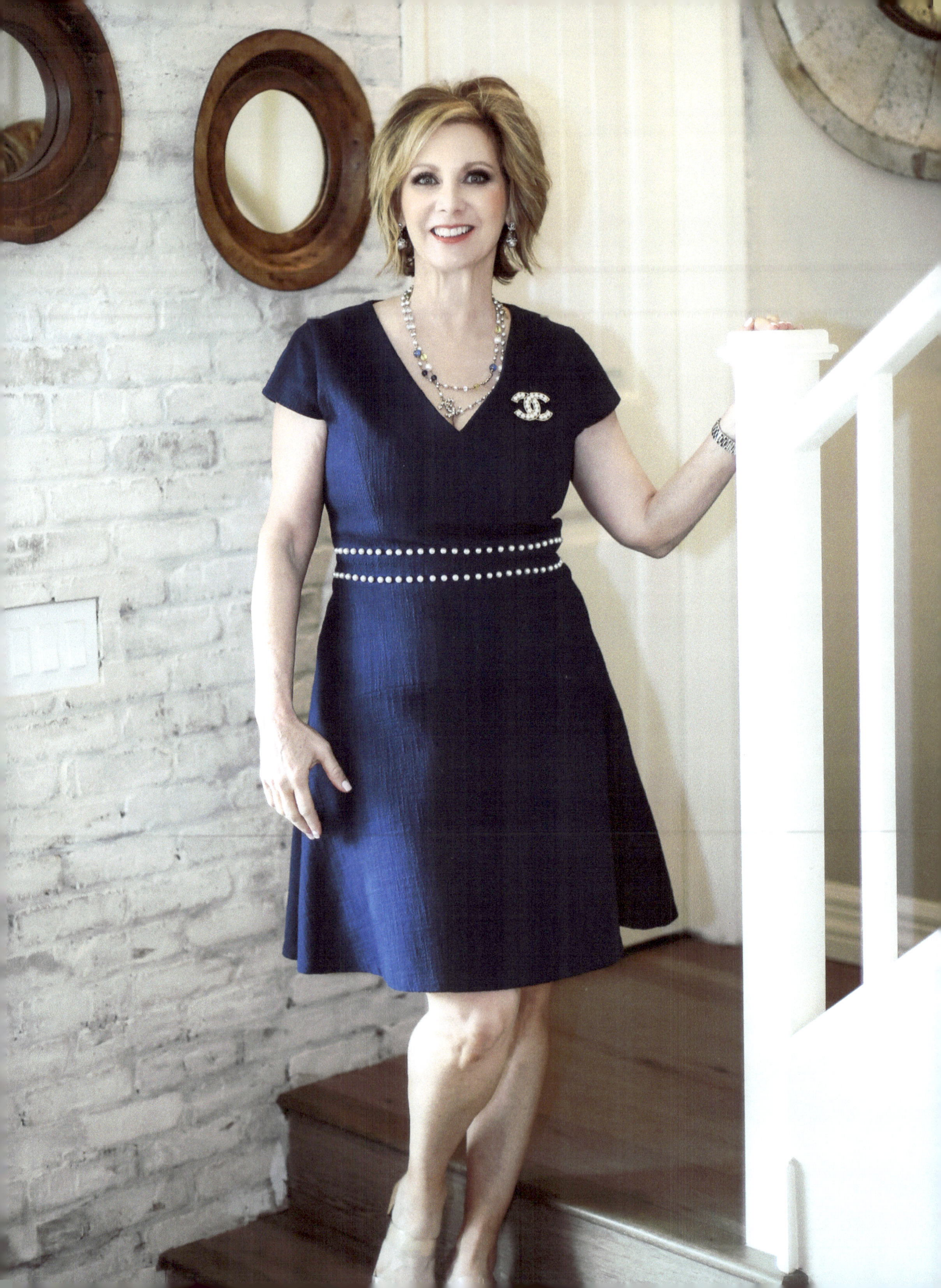

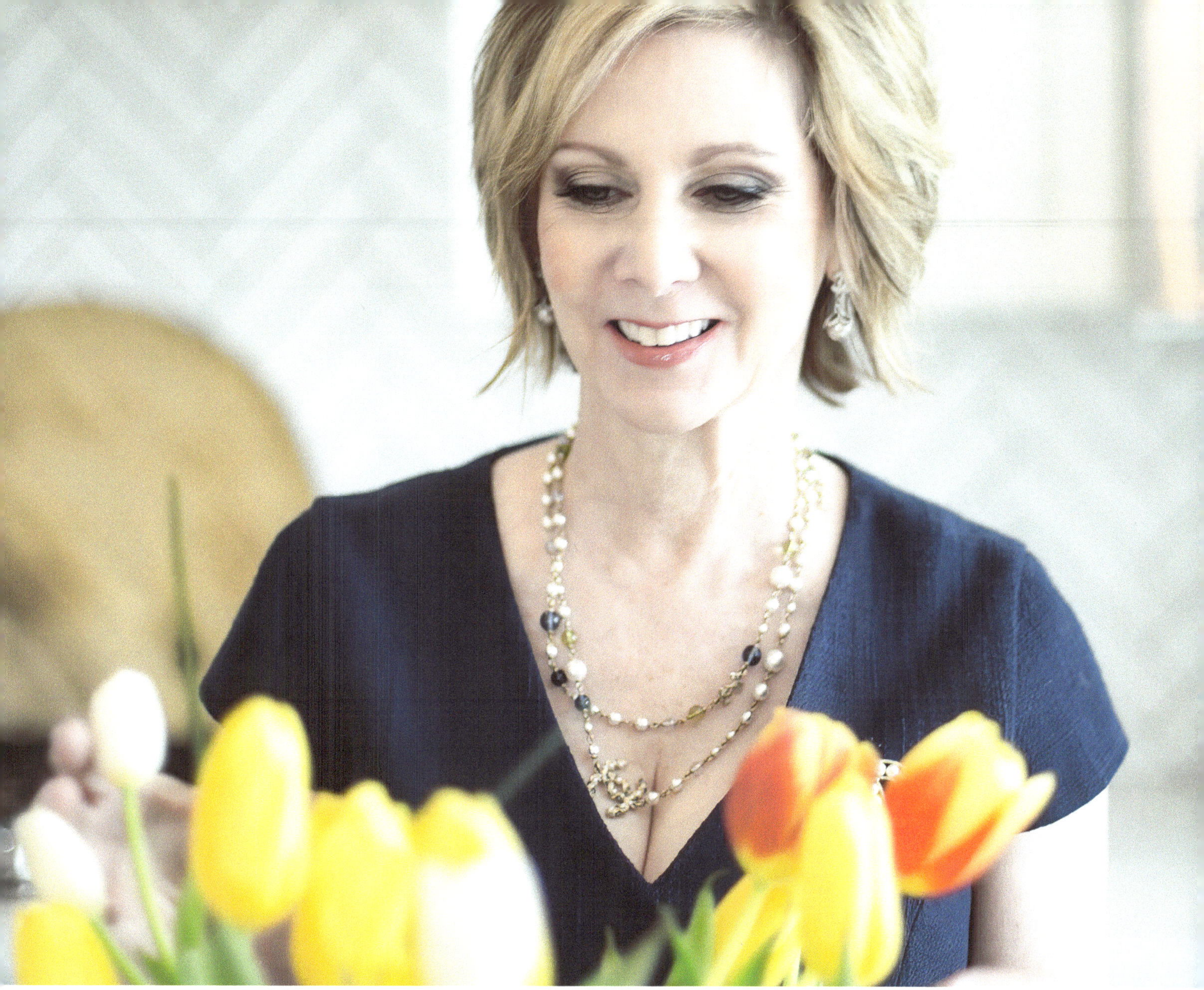

work or building my business. I am working on continuing this slower pace and being present in the moment.

How do you want to be remembered in your profession?

I want to be remembered as a pharmacist who cares about people! This was always the reason I wanted to become a pharmacist, people! My heart is truly filled with gratitude for the wonderful people I have met along the way in my career.

What's next for you and/or your business?

While I initially started ditchbladderpain.com , to empower women to gain freedom from bladder pain; the scope of what I share has reached to also include overactive bladder and urinary tract infections. I have recently studied holistic herbalism. I will be including an integrative approach to wellness that includes herbs as well in what I share with women. I truly want women to know that they can not only overcome bladder issues but look and feel their absolute best despite their diagnosis. A diagnosis may describe one's current health situation, but it does not define their life!

Where can we find you to further connect?

You can reach me at:

www.instagram.com/thefulfilledpharmacist

www.ditchbladderpain.com

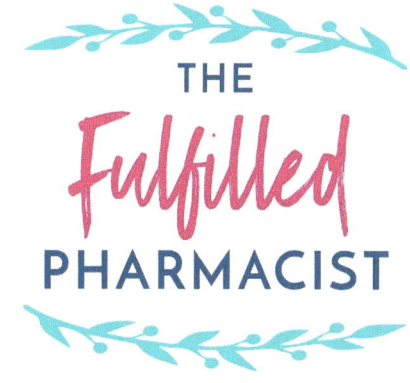

The Elevate Beachfront Retreat!
November 5-7, 2021!

A transformative 3-day luxury retreat for visionary pharmacist entrepreneurs ready to release blocks to amplify your income & impact!

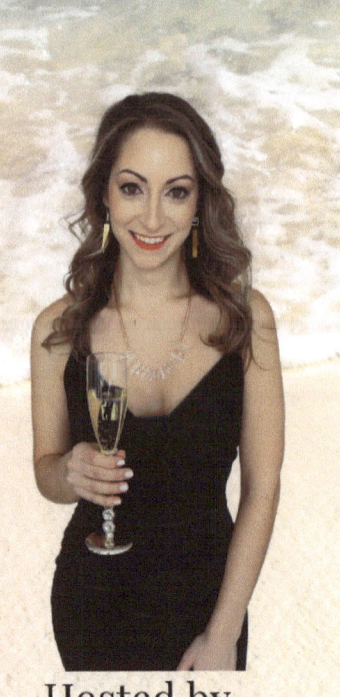

Hosted by -
Dr. Christina Fontana
The Pharmacist Coach™

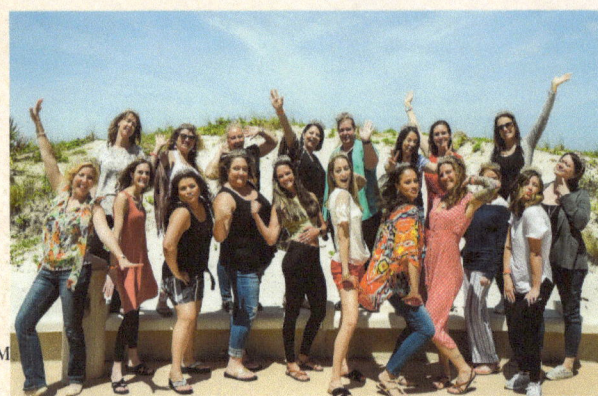

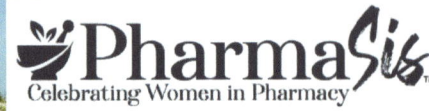

Media Partner – PharmaSis™ Magazine

Are you a pharmacist entrepreneur looking to Elevate your Business?
Join us at The November Elevate Retreat!

A transformative 3-day luxury retreat for visionary pharmasist's to release blocks holding you back so you can elevate to your next level of income & impact!

Hosted by Dr. Christina Fontana
The Pharmacist Coach™

Media partner – PharmaSis™ Magazine

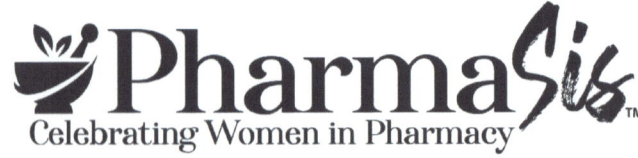

The November Elevate Retreat!

A 3-day luxury immersion experience for visionary pharmacist entrepreneurs ready to...

- Release blocks holding you back so you can **elevate to YOUR next level in your business!**
- Learn powerful tools and strategies to connect to your heart to **accelerate the path to your big vision!**
- Clear fears, overwhelm, doubt, and self-sabotage and **anchor in UNSHAKEABLE confidence!**
- Claim your authentic VOICE and self-expression to **show up as the powerful Queen you are!**
- Tap into your soul gifts, raise your energy, and **elevate your income and impact!**
- Take your power back and **own your light out in the world!**

Claim your ticket for Elevate through the link below!

www.bitly.com/elevatefallretreat

Use coupon code **PHARMASIS** for $200 off the ticket price!

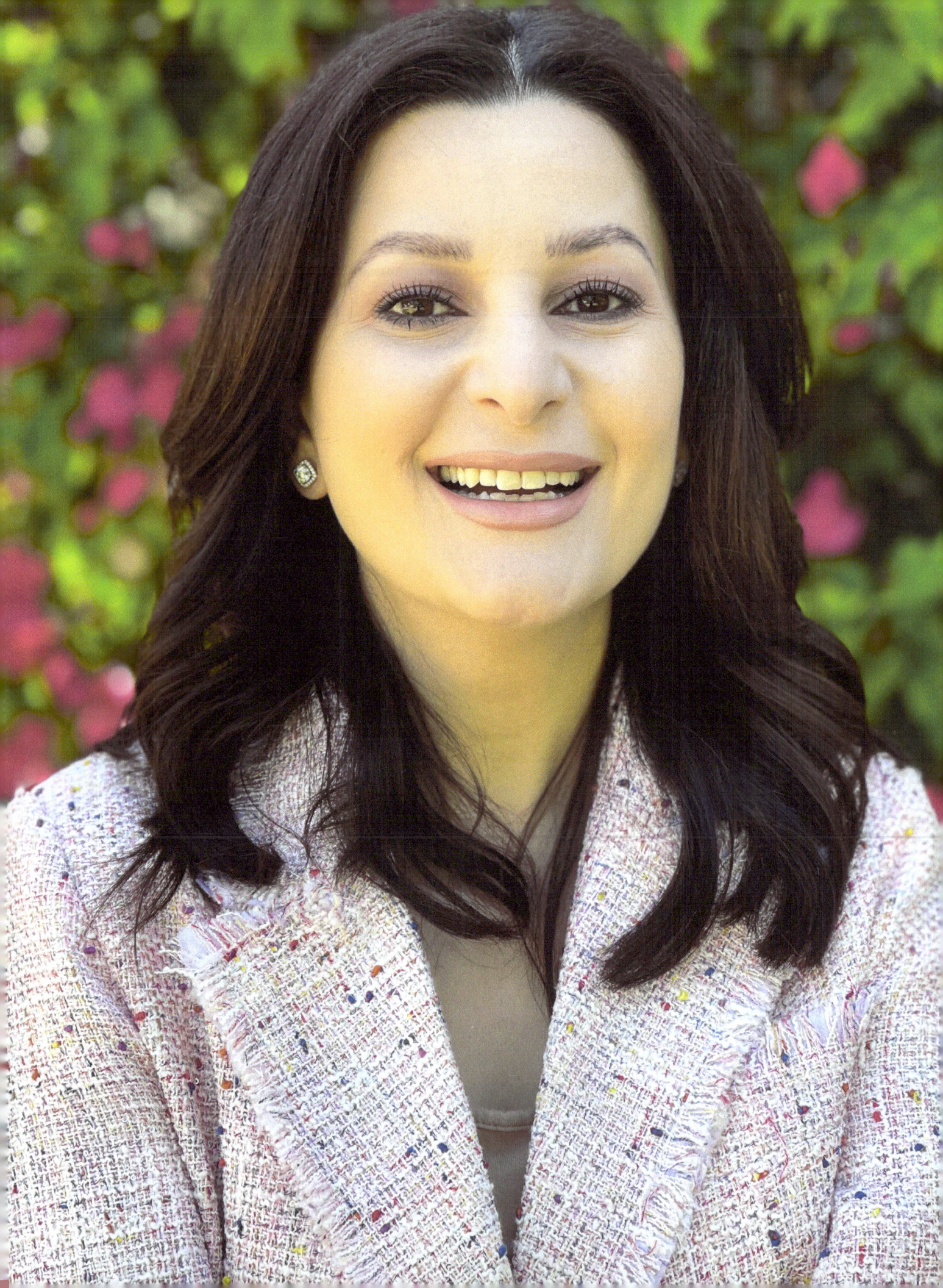

PHARMACOGENOMICS

DR. ANI ROSTOMYAN
living life fearlessly

LOS ANGELES, CA | PHARMACY SCHOOL: **YEREVAN STATE MEDICAL UNIVERSITY, MASSACHUSETTS COLLEGE OF PHARMACY AND HEALTH SCIENCES** | DEGREES: **MASTER'S DEGREE IN PHARMACY, PHARMD** | PREVIOUS CAREER: **COMMUNITY PHARMACIST** | NOW CAREER: **AMBULATORY CARE PHARMACIST, PHARMACOGENOMICS CONSULTANT PHARMACIST, DIABETES EDUCATOR**

Tell your story…how did you get here?

'If you always do what you always did, you'll always get what you always got" - *Henry Ford.*

I grew up in a very traditional Armenian family, where my father was the Patriarch of the family and we had held ourselves to very high standards in education and society. I am the youngest in the family and had learned to follow the lead from a young age.

The programming I grew up with was to follow your superior's direction and always be the best employee you can, he would always say small and steady income is always better than risky entrepreneurial ventures and taking risks is not smart. He was a follower himself and never infused confidence in his daughters as well.

My father passed away from Diabetes complications in 2010 at the age of 69, which is the reason I am passionate about Diabetes education and empowering my patients to feel and be more in charge of their health.

The detrimental effects of childhood programming sadly grew stronger in me in adulthood as well. I was expected to be an excellent mother, wife, professional, homemaker and not be allowed to feel overwhelmed.

Frankly, that discipline helped me in some way, with English as my second language, I succeeded to pass all my Foreign Pharmacist exams, get licensed in State of Florida and find my first pharmacist job so my Father would be proud of me.

Not until in my late 30's, having to move to California, after a divorce, now as a single mother, working as a Clinical Pharmacist, I realized that following was not something I felt empowered with, being a foreign graduate Pharmacist, I constantly felt the need to accomplish more and more every year.

Human psychology is a peculiar thing, people who succeed in their endeavors are not smarter than others, which I had to discover later on, it's just their dreams are so much bigger than the fear that's holding them back.

Fast forward to a Pandemic year, 2020, I broke my usual pattern of the follower, doer, overachiever, and fearlessly dove into self-developing more to an entrepreneur mindset and was astonished how much I loved it.

I established my own company SheAni, Inc, which resembles the fearless Ani, who is not afraid to go out of her way to make a difference in patients' lives and is not afraid to look brave and independent.

Describe what you are building/have built.

I established my consulting business and I am helping community Pharmacies to incorporate Pharmacogenomics as part of their MTM services, I also consult and assist physicians in ordering and interpreting Pharmacogenomic testing for patients.

What's been the biggest surprise about your recent journey?

The biggest surprise I encountered was that medical society is in dire need of Pharmacists as educators, leaders, and patient advocates. We don't only fill Doctors' orders; we help physicians tailor therapy to each and every patient's unique genomic profile and epigenetics. Pharmacists are obligated to own the Pharmacogenomics field as drug experts and take on the role of the indispensable part of the patient success team.

What is/was your biggest fear and how did you face it?

I faced the indescribable fear of leaving my comfort zone yet another time, but in such a different way, that led me to doubt many times the righteousness of the journey I was undertaking, and becoming the CEO of my own company, the decision maker and my own cheerleader.

What is your response to failure?

Our journey to success is hardly ever a linear road. I encourage others to acknowledge and talk about rejections and failures, not any less than emphasizing achievements. For example, I always tell the stories of how I failed my first attempt at the California CPJE exam, or my first failure of BCPS exam, and it is ok, I learned more and succeeded, it is never a sign of weakness to acknowledge that we didn't achieve our plans at first time.

What wisdom have you acquired that you would share with your younger self about your career journey?

I would advise the 20-year-old Ani not to fear disappointing others, and living the life I feel most in harmony, and look to find the ikigai that suits me, and no one else.

By what leadership principle do you lead yourself and others?

Leadership has many shades, there are quiet and outspoken leaders, or a mixture of both. I tend to be the quiet one, that leads by example and sincere advice, rather than extroverted approaches. I learned long ago, from my swimming instructor at a very young age, you can't just tell people not to be afraid of water and just jump, everyone learns differently, and leaders should recognize the personality types before becoming influencers.

What would you say to a woman who is unhappy in her current pharmacy role?

I say, you got this girlfriend!

Sometimes we have to adjust to many uncomfortable situations, including unfulfilling, unrewarding jobs, but utilizing the income from the current role in self-development is very beneficial and being productive while holding a full time career is an acceptable reality as well.

How are you getting back to business in life or business now that we seem to be adjusting to life during the pandemic?

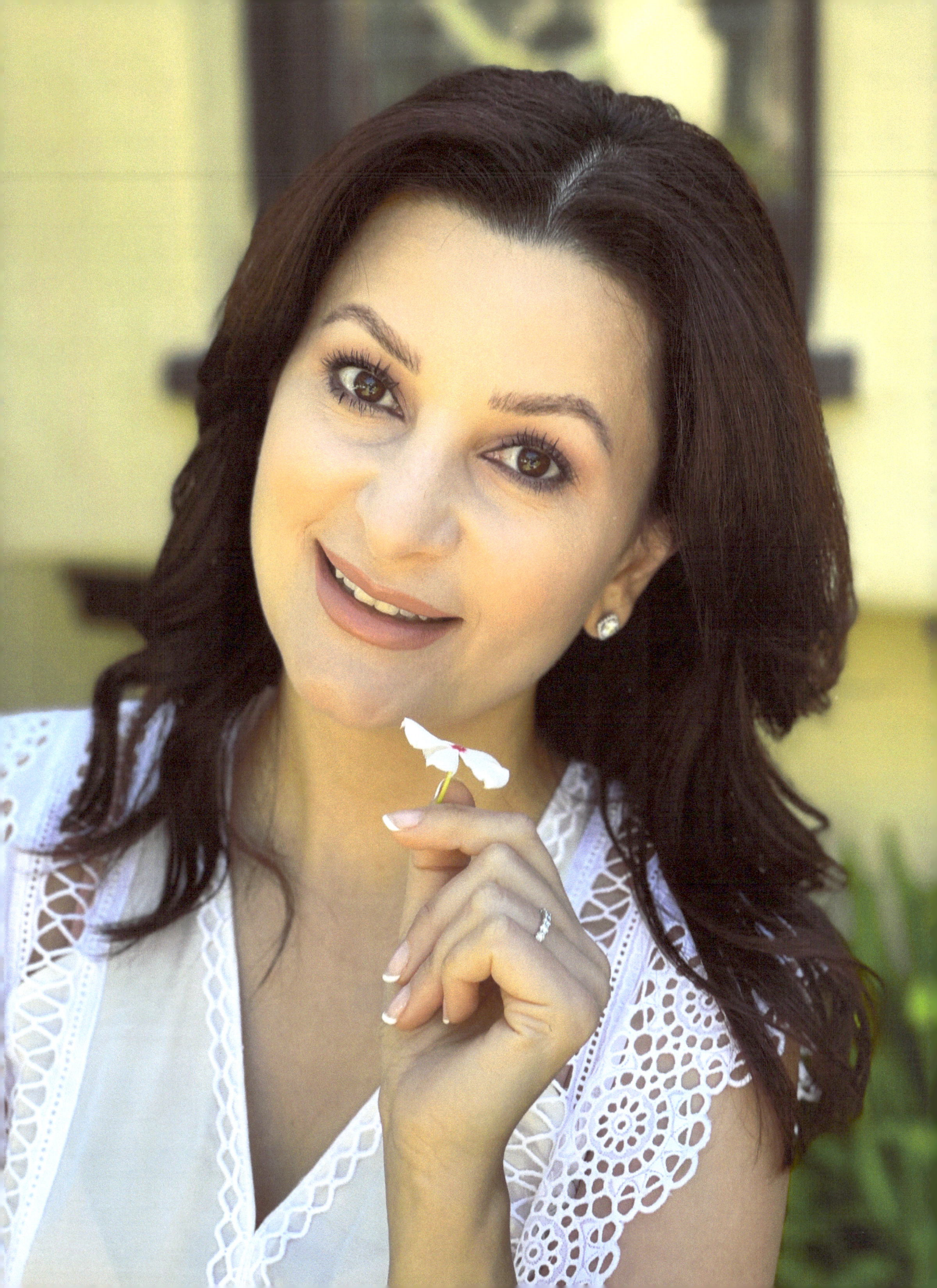

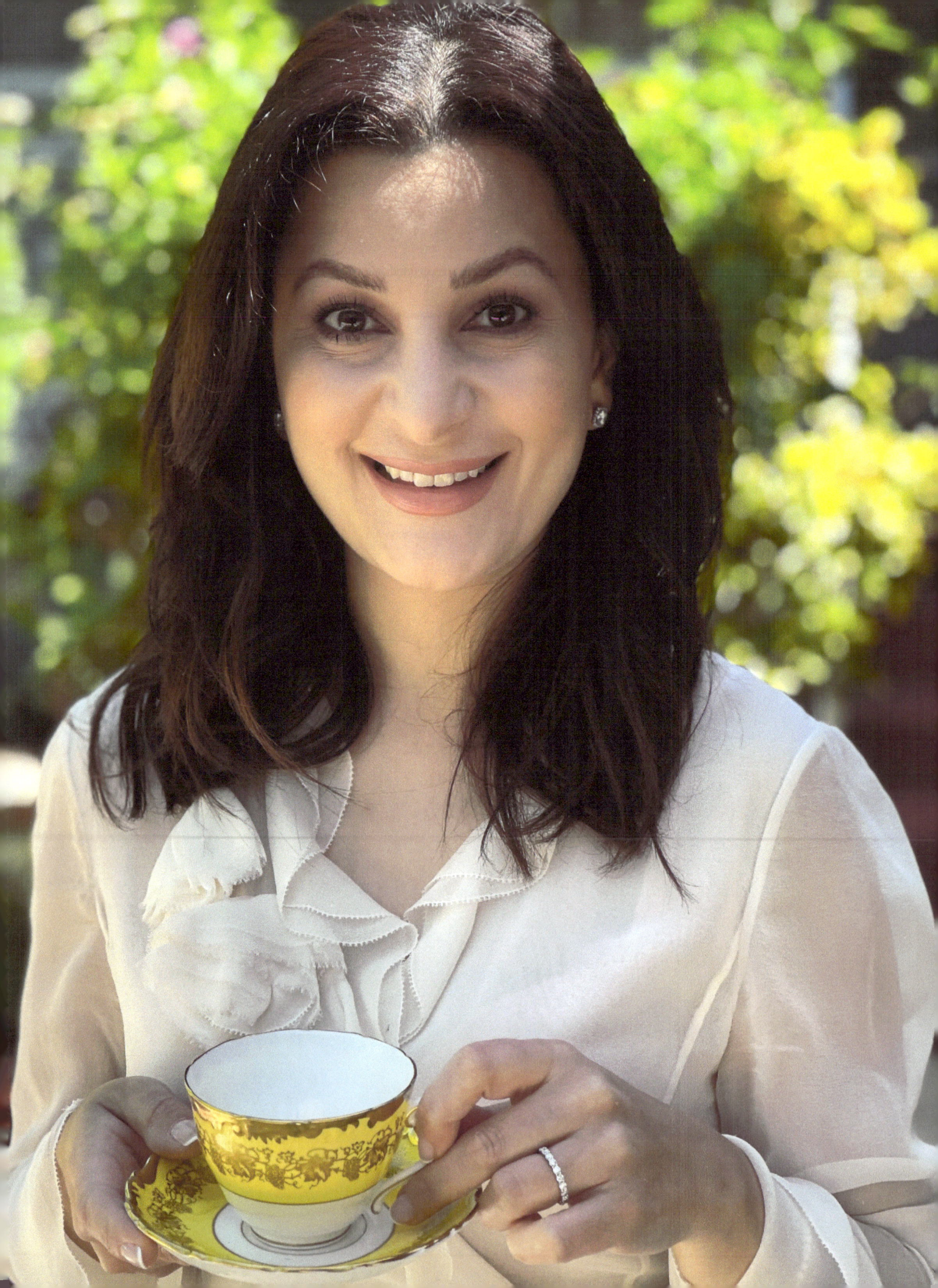

I feel like recovering from a longtime illness, gaining senses back step by step, first trying to create strategies to adjust to new realms in healthcare and developing business plans accordingly.

How do you want to be remembered in your profession?

I feel that the Pharmacy profession is a great fit for compassionate multitaskers, and if I changed the lives of patients for the better and improved their health outcomes; I feel accomplished.

I would like to be remembered as a pharmacist and a health coach that cared and went out of her way to help people with their unique health needs.

What is next for you and/or your business?

There's much going on in business development and more in person events are planned, thankfully!

I am partnering with a wonderful group of likeminded Pharmacists and creating much needed concierge Pharmacy consulting services and am very excited about this journey.

Where can we find you to further connect? (no email addresses or phone numbers please)

I do have a Linkedin page and business Instagram account for further connecting, please feel free to reach to me with questions and inquiries!

Instagram:

https://www.instagram.com/dr.anirostomyan/

Linked In:

linkedin.com/in/dr-ani-rostomyan-pharmd-bcps-aph-4885b622

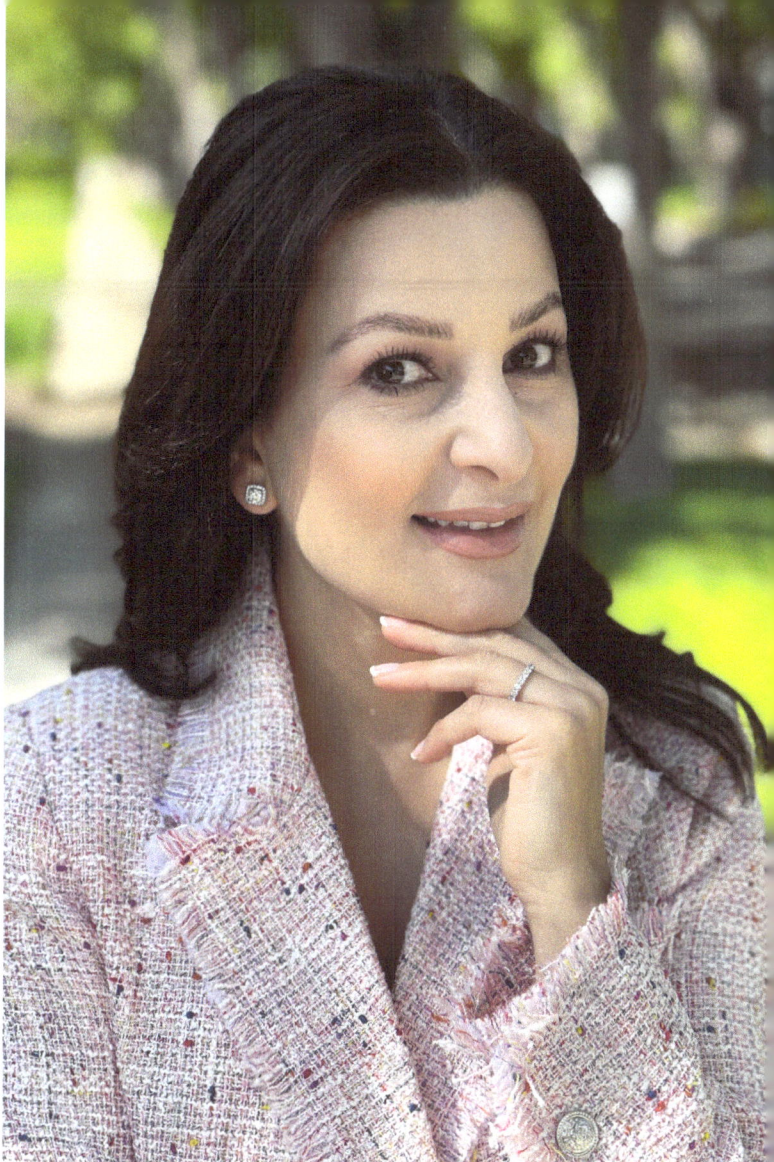

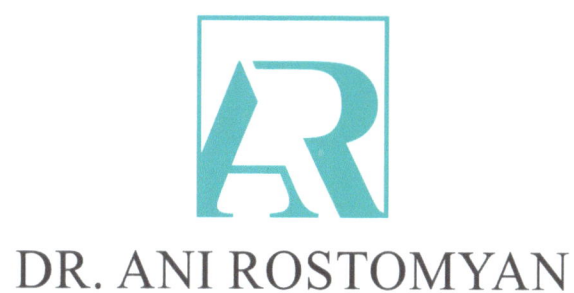

www://dranirostomyan.com

*"Old keys don't open new doors.
Do all things differently; if you have the confidence; if not, build."*
-unknown

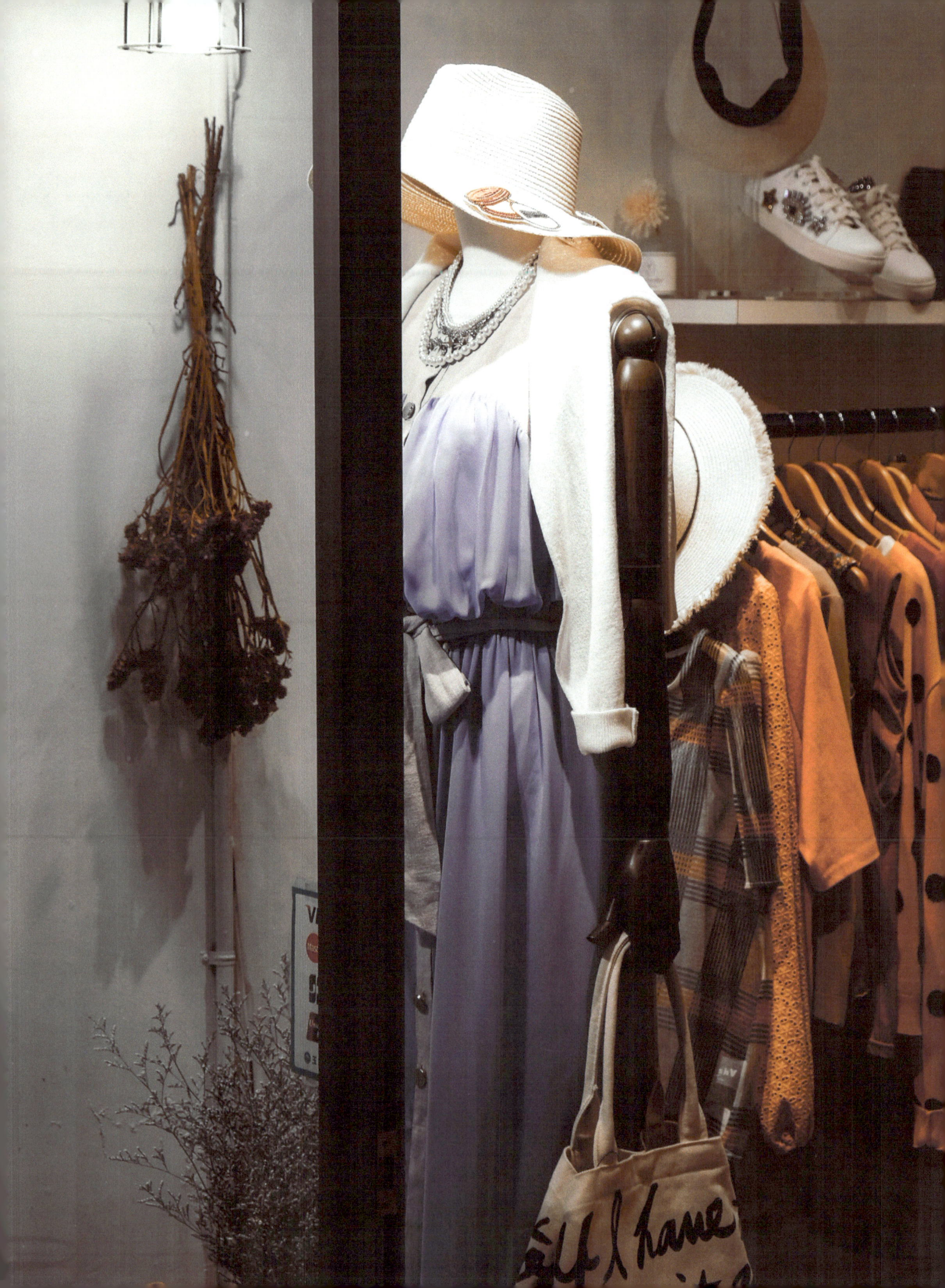

COVER STORY

style matters

Written by: Dr. Danielle Perrodin, *Contributing Author*

Style can be defined best as knowing who you are and what looks great on you. Recently I learned about the Enclothed Cognitive Theory from a style course I was enrolled in. My instructor had left medical school to pursue a more creative career helping women define their style and embody confidence. In the medical field, we are brought up to only trust evidence supported information. This is the conclusion made by Hajo Adam and Adam D. Galinsky: "Clothes systematically influence wearers' psychological processes."

The study found that the clothes you wear send messages to yourself and to others. Here are just a few examples of this:

• Formal clothing = Authoritative and powerful
• Casual clothing = Open and agreeable
• Active wear = Works out and healthy

Changing the clothes that you wear is just one easy way to embody the woman you want to become. You can begin dressing as she would dress if she already had the results that you currently desire. This will allow you to change your belief system of what is possible for you, now. Decide who you want to be and how you want to be perceived. Curate the wardrobe that supports this.

When you look good, you feel good and treat others better. Not only will you treat others better, but you will treat yourself better. You may work out more, market yourself more consistently on social media and/or attend more networking events in person. By raising your confidence level and self-esteem, you will begin to hold your head up, shoulders back, and make eye contact. The clothes you wear affect how you carry yourself. This body language is a form of non-verbal communication. This will improve all relationships in your life and business.

Style tells a story. It sends out messages. It impacts your confidence and self-esteem. Your thoughts about yourself and the clothes you wear do in fact impact your mood and how you feel which translates into the actions you take and ultimately the results and reality you create. To create a reality you choose on purpose, purposefully choose your wardrobe. One of the best ways to do this is to hire a qualified and objective person such as style and image coach like myself. Now that you realize how style matters, begin improving your style today, one step at a time.

Dr. Danielle Perrodin, Integrative Style & Image Coach and Behavioral Health/LTC Pharmacist. My mission is to help women create happier, healthier more beautiful lives. Through integrating the mind, body and spirit, my clients expedite the time it takes to close the gap between their highest authentic self (who they truly are) and how they appear to the world. I combine my love for fashion and coaching to give my clients unique tools to style their mind and body in order to learn how to Be Her(£) Now!

I have had the pleasure of styling Dr. Lauren Castle, Founder of FmPhA who was featured in Katie Couric Media and Dr. Kristine Cline, both previously featured in PharmaSis Magazine.

Married to Kevin for 19 years, we currently reside in south Louisiana with our twin boys, Ethan and Landon, and daughter Mori Lee. I learned early on that life is too short when I lost my step daughter Megan and first love Joey in separate car crashes. They all are the reasons I do what I do. Memento Mori.

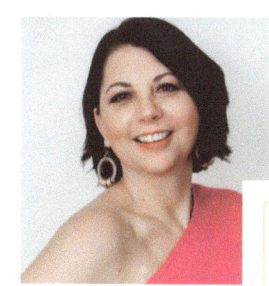

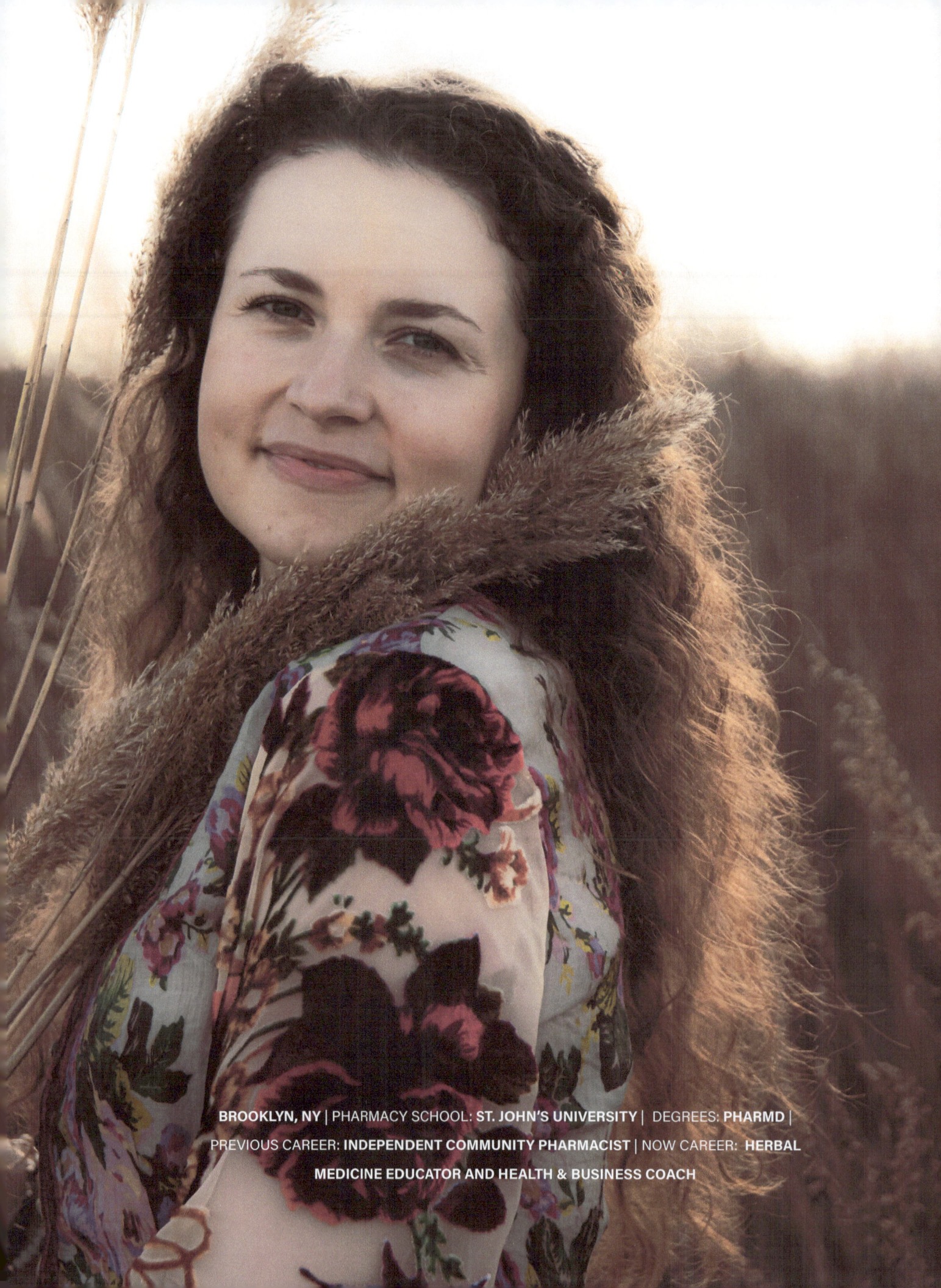

BROOKLYN, NY | PHARMACY SCHOOL: **ST. JOHN'S UNIVERSITY** | DEGREES: **PHARMD** | PREVIOUS CAREER: **INDEPENDENT COMMUNITY PHARMACIST** | NOW CAREER: **HERBAL MEDICINE EDUCATOR AND HEALTH & BUSINESS COACH**

HERBAL MEDICINE EDUCATOR

Dr. Marina Buksov

Helping Women Thrive

Tell your story…how did you get here?

When I was graduating pharmacy school in 2013, I was at a complete loss as to what I actually want to do with my degree and skill set. I realized I'm actually not passionate about any of the coveted and highly competitive options I was interviewing for. I was having serious psychosomatic symptoms, that at the time I didn't identify as such. I was feeling nauseous, having weird burping, and had constant tearing from both eyes. I also realized right around this time that I'm not with the right life partner, and broke up with my boyfriend of six years.

Things just kept getting worse, as I tried various modalities, followed the advice of various professionals, and changed my diet. I thought I was doing the healthy and responsible things, but kept getting worse. Going vegan and drinking raw green smoothies seemed to exacerbate my symptoms, and I kept gaining weight and my periods started getting irregular. I started to break out in angry red blisters all over my face, though I always had clear skin as a teen.

I found the gentle natural healing approach after personally suffering trauma from excessive overmedicalization and invasive treatment with allopathic methods. From gastrointestinal distress (irritable bowel syndrome), to overgrowth of stomach and gut bacteria, to adult onset acne, to a mysterious inflammatory eye condition, I was no stranger at various medical facilities and doctors' offices. I even frequented various alternative practitioners such as energy healers, acupuncturists, craniosacral therapists and herbalists.

Through this whole journey, I lost twice what I paid in rent to twice-weekly out of pocket sessions with an energy worker, with no improvement in a year. I raised my intraocular pressure by following the prescribed doses of local steroidal drops into my eyes. I underwent general anesthesia in order to have a surgical procedure done involving a temporary stent placement in my tear duct. And I earned two black eye fiascos, by way of acupuncture and aggressive manual irrigation of my left eye, respectively.

I've agreed to various diagnostic procedures, rigorous testing, polypharmacy, and elective surgeries, and paid out of pocket for many interventions…and found no relief whatsoever. All of my trials and tribulations led me to find that there's a better way. Through my own process of addressing gut health, focusing on whole foods and herbs, and creating space in my life for spirit and joy, I've found the way to true holistic health.

Professionally, I got to this point where I had a deep internal conflict. I'd have an inner dialogue to justify my career path to myself, but felt powerless to change it. Although a very coveted and respected field in my circle of friends and family, I found myself feeling resentful and ashamed. I hated what I did on a day to day basis: hand out huge bags of pharmaceutical medications on doctors' orders. I felt that I was doing a disservice by playing this tiny role in a hugely flawed medical system.

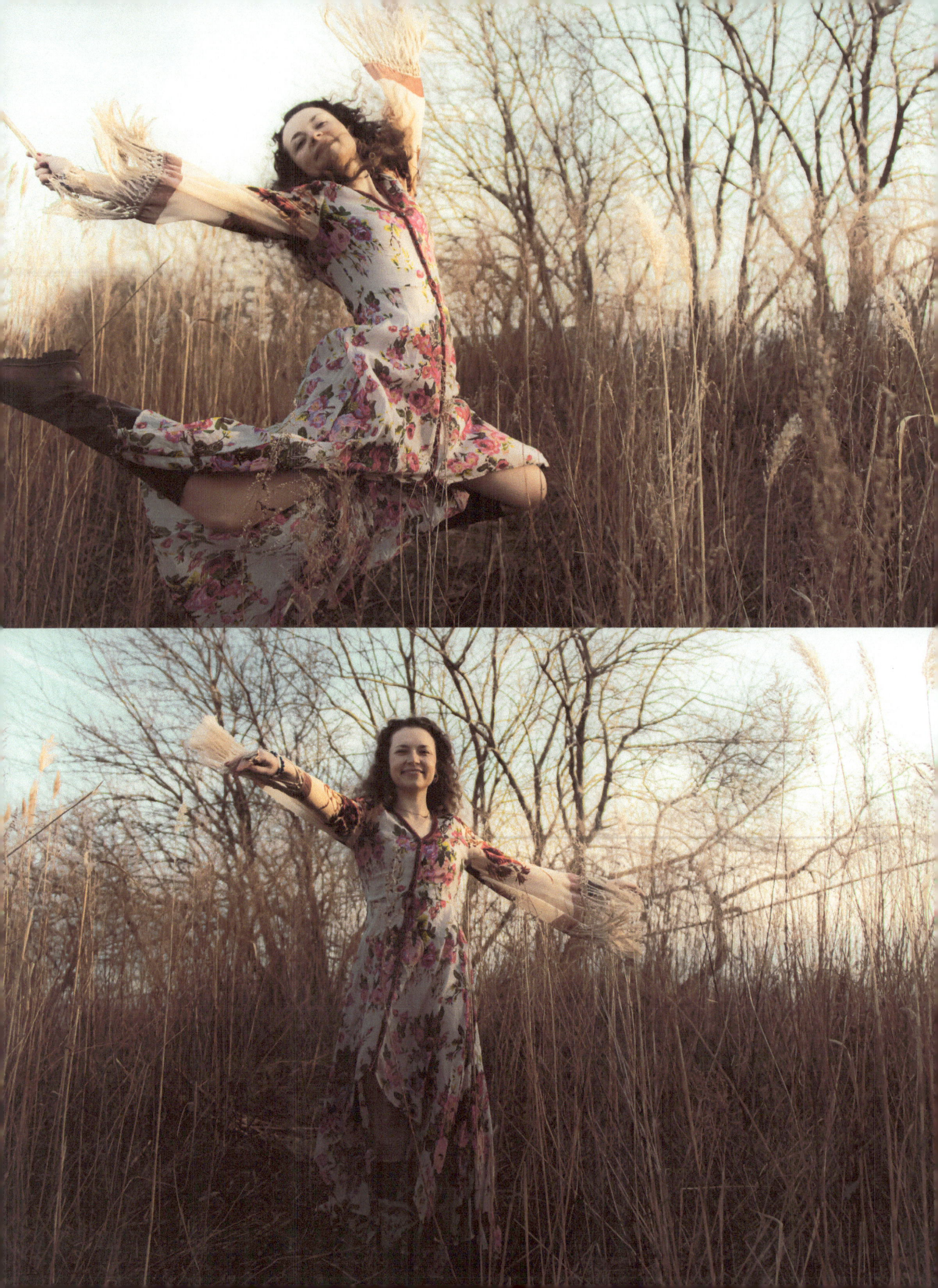

My heart was wrenched because I felt, and knew firsthand, that my nonpharmacological expertise can help people reduce medication burden, improve symptoms, and boost health and vitality. However, I had neither the time to offer advice, nor was there much interest among my patients to invest in methods that were not covered by their health insurance plan.

In addition, I could not help but notice all the waste that was involved in every step of the pharmacy business, from production, to shipping, to dispensing. I could only imagine a landline continually filling with billions of plastic stock as well as individual prescription bottles. Not to mention all the paper and other garbage we accumulate on a daily basis, with little regard for recycling in some workplaces.

I wanted to find a way to use my background and education as a pharmacist to be a positive influence, and contribute to building a better society of tomorrow in a sustainable and eco-conscious manner. But I had no idea how to start over, or how to apply myself better. And I didn't want to admit that all my schooling and efforts, all the fruit of my parents' and my labors, were in vain. That I invested so much time, work and money into a dream that didn't fulfill me.

Fast forward through various trainings and continuing my education in the fields of health coaching, functional nutrition, functional medicine, and clinical herbalism - today I am a small business owner as a consultant and educator. I am an advocate for getting the least invasive, most gentle approach to both diagnosis and treatment. I help to support and activate one's own body's innate healing mechanisms using lifestyle modalities, and whole foods & herbs. I believe health and happiness are really a way of looking at and living life; rather than a particular destination that we often seek. Additionally, I educate and train other health care professionals to expand their income & impact through holistic herbal medicine.

Describe what you are building/have built (your business)

I have recently launched my first retreat, called La Raiz ("the root" in Spanish) - an invitation to bridge together ancient tradition and wisdom with the current healthcare model. This will supplement my main online 6-month immersion into Herbalism program, which is a comprehensive guide to integrate herbalism into an existing practice or start a brand new business with the tools I teach.

(https://www.drmarinabuksov.com/services/build-your-holistic-herbal-practice/)

I also see patients via the telehealth platform, PharmToTable - using my diverse background through the lens of functional medicine.

What's been the biggest surprise about your recent journey?

The most surprising part of walking this entrepreneurial path is having to dive deep into mindset and personal development and face my own demons. Not only am I having to learn new skill sets in the business realm, but also level up in very real and personal ways at each step of the process. I have learned that I have been living with deep seated insecurities and fears, but that I'm also resilient and can learn new habits, if I want something bad enough. I have learned that you can't "have it all" - at one time. Each stage of the journey requires some sort of sacrifice, but at the end of each stage, my life feels more full and wholesome. It's all about prioritizing and reaching the "non-negotiable" goals first; and making time for the less "priority" goals by scheduling those in along the way. True fulfillment not only requires fierce determination, but also grace and surrender at times.

What is/was your biggest fear and how did you face it?

My biggest fear is that I won't make a difference in a positive way, that my voice won't be heard, that my efforts will be in vain. That I will be laughed at, misunderstood, judged, and my business will fail (and everyone will bear witness to this failure, and I may have to go beg for employment again). I face this fear daily and make the daily decision to keep going anyway, one step at a time. There is nothing else I'd rather do than at least TRY to live out what's in my heart. So I choose to speak my truth, go after what feels important for me, and solve one problem at a time.

What is your response to failure?

Taking personal responsibility for the factors over which I had control, and learning from my mistakes. Failure is really just a lesson, not a loss. The biggest failure of all is not taking any action, or giving up. Success only comes to those who are fiercely persistent and keep going, despite failures.

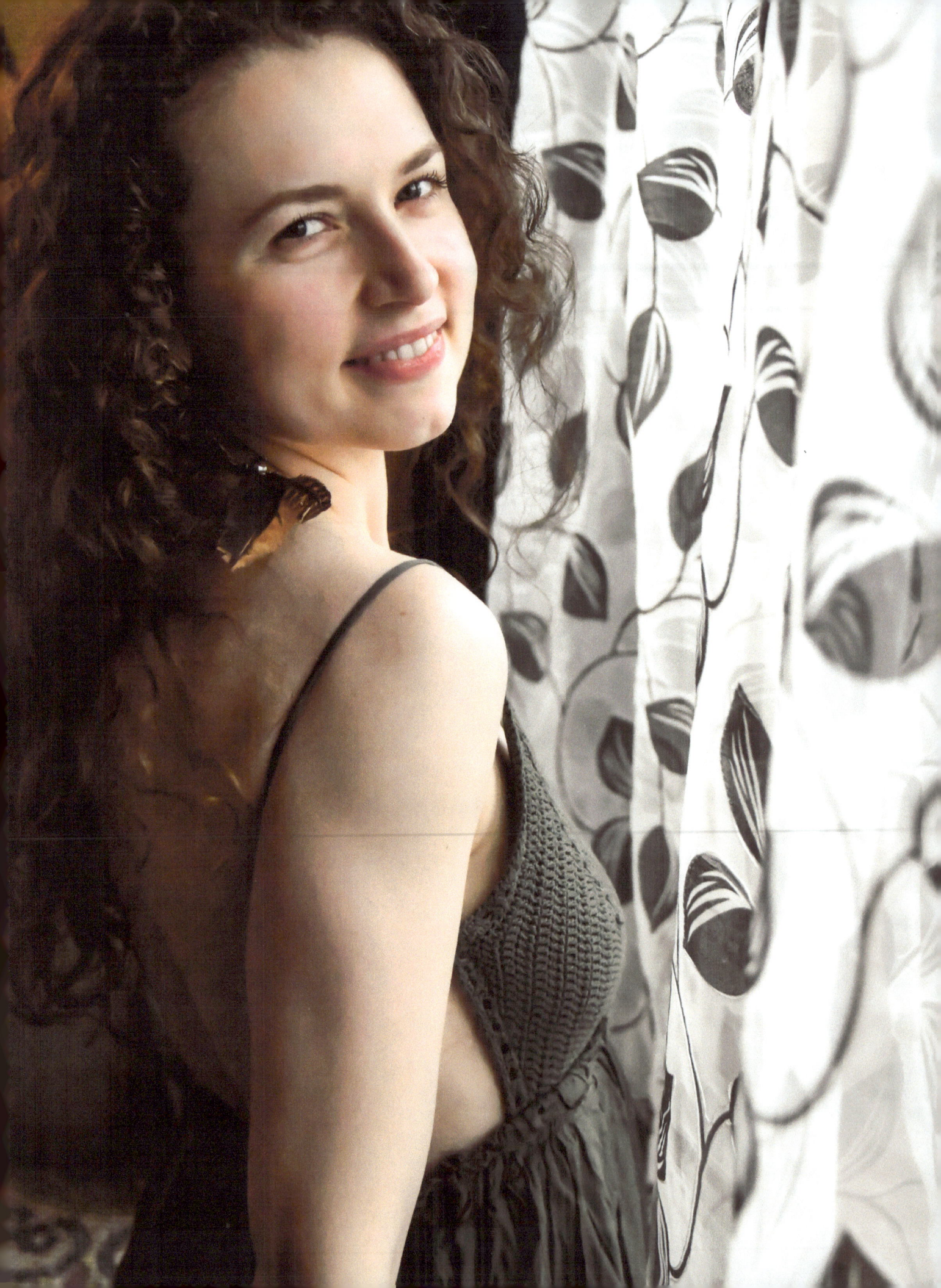

What wisdom have you acquired that you would share with your younger self about your career journey?

Have faith, listen to your own inner compass, and don't be afraid to fail. Walk away from what doesn't serve you, and leap into what makes your heart sing. Make space in your life for stillness, reflection, rest and creativity. Lead with your wildest dreams, and focus on what you want, in order for these things to have a chance at manifesting. Don't wait, and don't waste time on regrets; the perfect time is now.

By what leadership principle do you lead yourself and others?

Inspiring myself by role models, getting coached by mentors that I can relate to and have gone through a similar journey and came out on the other side. I share my passion and vision with others who resonate and help them cut the learning curve.

What would you say to a woman who is unhappy in her current pharmacy role?

You always have a choice. You are not under lock and key, nor a prisoner of your former decisions. Each day is another opportunity to make a different decision and to formulate a new plan, and set yourself up for the future of your dreams. You owe it to yourself, and to others who are looking up to you (including your kids, family, friends, colleagues, etc.) to be that change you wish to see. You have one life (that we know of), so make sure you're calling the shots and living it as you see fit.

How are you getting back to business in life or business now that we seem to adjusting to life during the pandemic?

I spent the better part of the pandemic working in an independent community pharmacy setting, and my whole family got COVID (thankfully, only suffered a light form of the illness). Now I'm starting a brand new chapter going full time into my business, and 100% remote work. After my retreat, I'll be focusing on my 6 month course that I'm offering to other healthcare professionals who are interested in building their holistic herbal practices. And I will still see patients remotely via the PharmToTable functional medicine platform.

How do you want to be remembered in your profession?

I want to be seen as a visionary who brings back something that was lost in pharmacy practice. I believe a pharmacist is a bridge between sick care and health care, that we can educate and empower patients about being their own advocate, and allowing them to take charge not only of their health journey, but their life. Health is so multifaceted, and if we focus on prevention and self-care, we can really lessen the burden on the healthcare system, save billions of healthcare dollars spent, and come out with a happier and healthier population. We need to work as a team, with other providers and patients, to get to the root causes of the problems that affect most areas of health. Tackling those will have a domino downstream effect. I would like to be seen as a pharmacist who can point to the least invasive, less costly, and most natural methods to provide a holistic solution for my patients. Our pharmacies don't have to be product-oriented, but health-outcomes oriented. I believe nutrition, lifestyle, and herbal medicine can all be great tools to fill in the gaps in care, and can be part of pharmacy practice.

What's next for you and/or your business?

I will continue to offer my online 6-month immersion into Herbalism program, a comprehensive guide to integrate herbalism into an existing practice or start a brand new business with the tools I teach. I will also be teaching workshops and creating programs for non-healthcare professionals who want to incorporate herbalism into their families' lives. After I build out my online space and offerings, who knows - I may open a functional herbal product line and/or open a wellness or retreat center!

Where can we find you to further connect? (no email addresses or phone numbers please)

https://www.drmarinabuksov.com/
Podcast: https://www.drmarinabuksov.com/podcasts/
Youtube: https://bit.ly/HOLISTICPHARMACYFacebook: @rawfork
Instagram: @drmarinabuksov
Linked In: @marinabuksov
Book a call: https://calendly.com/rawfork

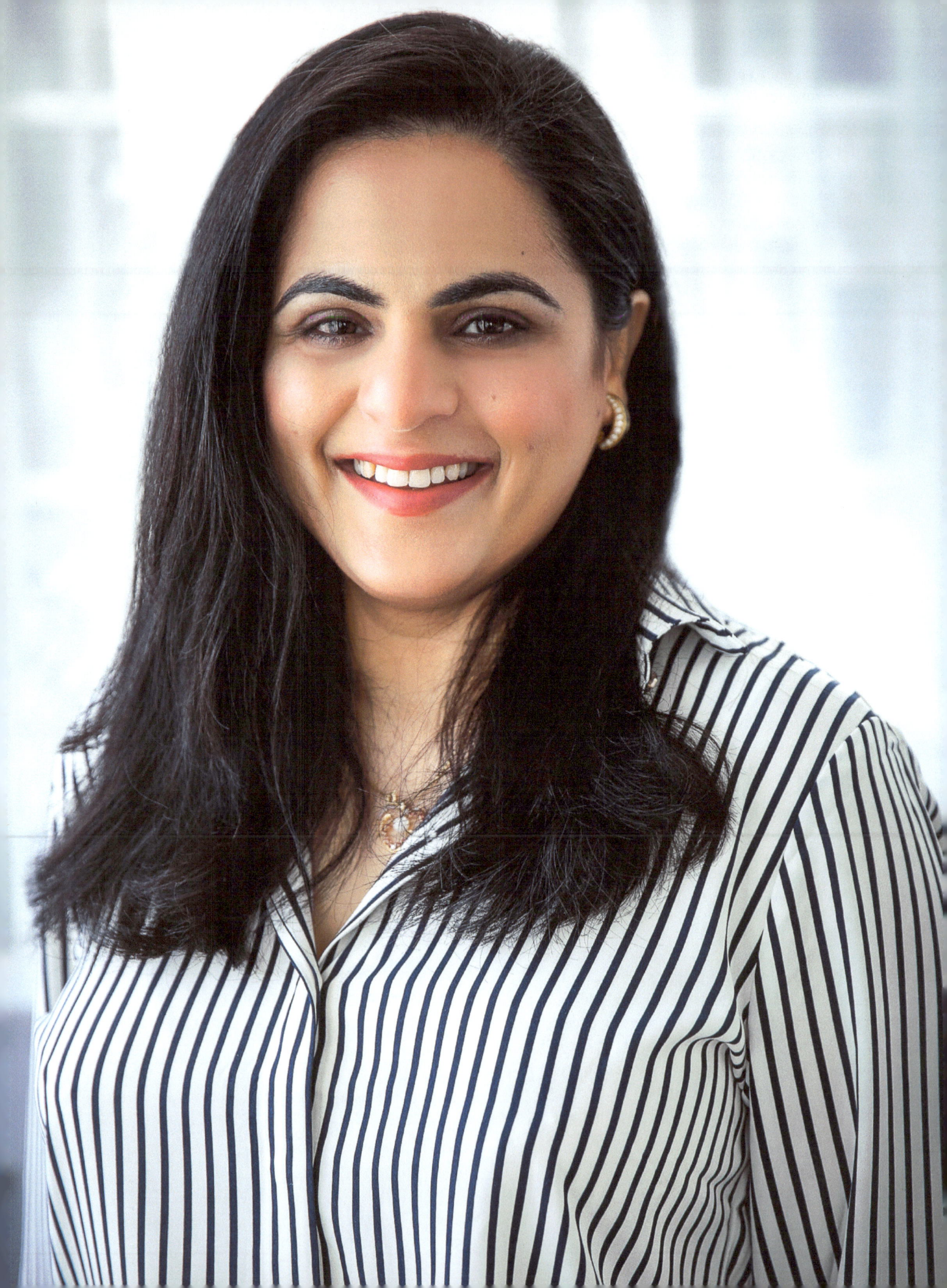

CONTRIBUTING AUTHOR SPOTLIGHT

Dr. Chinki Bhatia

Tell us a little about yourself

My name is Dr. Chinki Bhatia, I grew up in a small island called the kingdom of Bahrain. I'm a mother, consultant pharmacist and an avid follower of Ayurvedic living. In my spare time I love to kayak, hike and make good meals

Describe your passion and why it's important.

I Co- Founded my company Core Care Rx in January 2021 where I practice a holistic approach to preventing and managing diseases using innovative technologies such as pharmacogenomics, nutrigenomics, chronic care management and Ayurveda. What all of them have in common is their alignment with prevention rather than only treatment. This is exactly what I'm passionate about - I firmly believe that we must make prevention of disease and health promotion our priority in healthcare rather than just treatment.

What do you want women in pharmacy to take away from your expertise shared in your articles

The recent decade has witnessed many landmark observations, which has made the western world more receptive to eastern healthcare philosophy. However, Ayurveda (ancient Indian medicine) has been persistently criticised for it's ambiguity. Through my writing, I'd like to bridge the gap between Ayurveda and modern science and decode core concepts of Ayurveda that could be used and taught to improve one's health in daily life.

Tell us a fun fact about yourself:

I enjoy eating peanut butter, cucumber sandwiches rather than peanut butter with jelly!

How can readers connect with you?

www.corecarerx.com | Instagram: @corecarerx, Dr.Chinki Bhatia | Facebook @corecarerx

5 Invigorating Ayurvedic Drinks that Pharmacists can Endorse for Diabetic Patients!

Written by: Chinki Bhatia

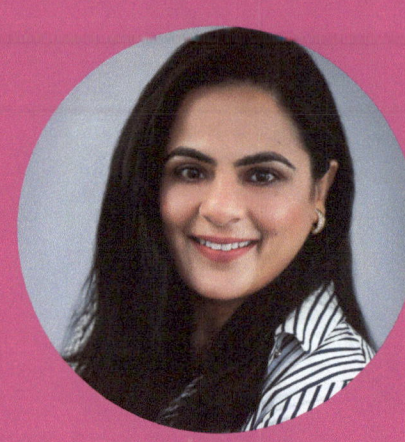

The overwhelming heat of summer is quickly approaching, and very soon we will be looking for cool drinks to beat the heat! But have you noticed that this generation often looks for quick fixes in the form of aerated and ready made packaged drinks containing sugar and preservatives? These drinks not only increase the risk for metabolic syndrome but also reduce the ability of people who already have diabetes to control blood glucose. Fortunately, Ayurveda offers recipes for many rejuvenating diabetic friendly summer drinks.

Ayurveda condemns the consumption of ice-cold foods and beverages, as they disrupt the digestive fire called Agni. However, it does encourage drinking cool beverages to lower one's body temperature and balance the Pitta Dosha. Cold water is great for this purpose, though there are other options Ayurveda recommends.

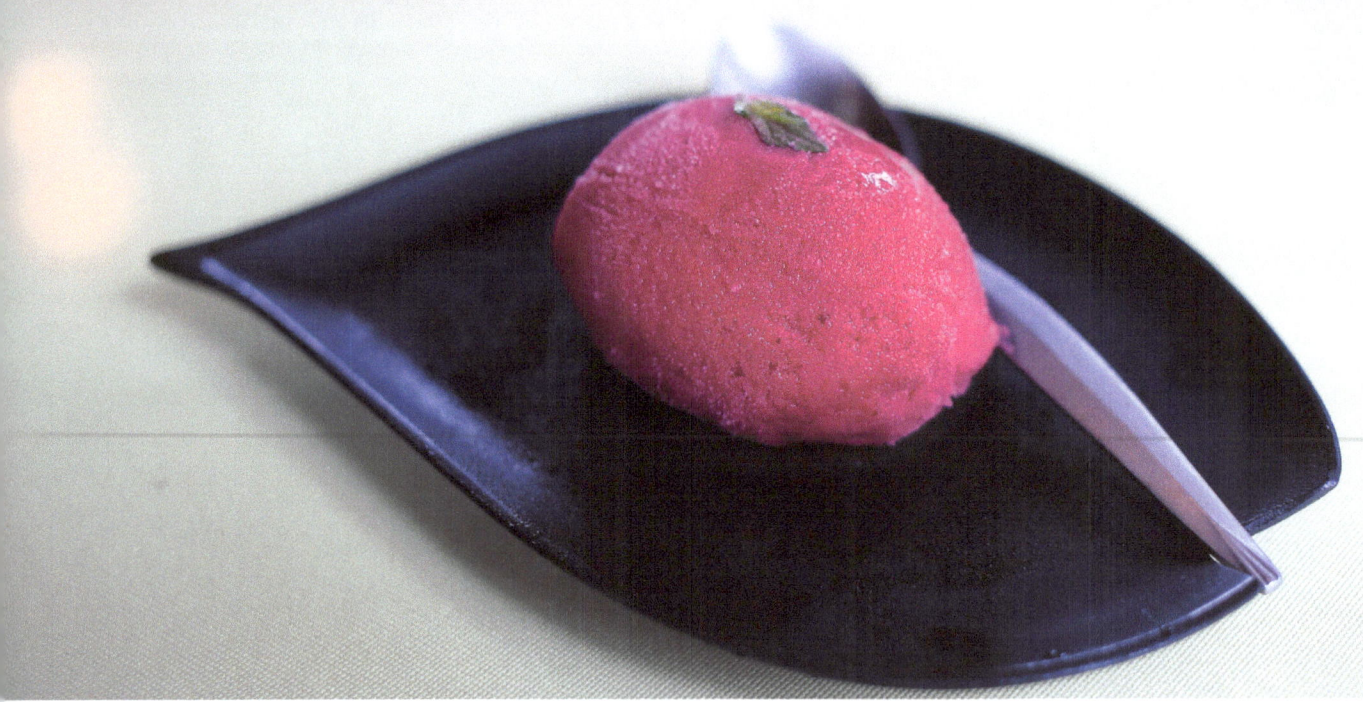

Here are 5 diabetic friendly drinks that Pharmacists can advise to their patients and physicians

Rose sherbet with sweet basil seeds reduces stress and anxiety due to its cooling properties. It contains no added sugar and is rich in fiber. The sweet basil seeds, are popular for their health benefits—for example, they help control blood sugar levels relieve digestive problems.

Ingredients: sugar- and preservative-free rose syrup, water, sweet basil seeds

Directions: Soak 1 tsp of basil seeds for a few minutes in ½ cup of water. Combine 2 tbsp of rose syrup, water, and ice in a cup. Add a few basil seeds and stir.

Sattu (roasted, powdered barley and gram pulses) is an age-old potent Indian drink that is all-natural, rich in fiber and protein, and loaded with iron and magnesium. It has a very low glycemic index, and so it won't cause your blood sugar levels to spike. This makes it a diabetic-friendly food!

Ingredients: Store-bought organic barely gram flour, water, rock salt, ice

Directions: Blend 2 tbsp of gram flour with one cup of water. Add ice and rock salt.

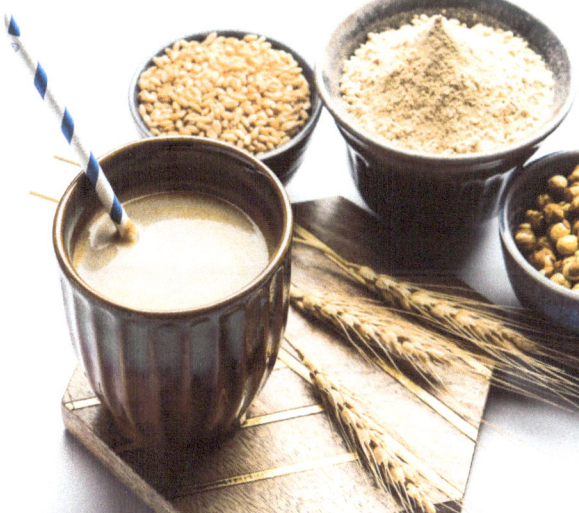

Traditional buttermilk is made from the liquid leftover from whole milk that's been churned into butter. Buttermilk can be mixed with water and tempered with curry leaves, fenugreek and mustard seeds to improve its probiotic, digestive, and blood-sugar-lowering effects. This all-rounder is surely a perfect solution to your summer woes.

Ingredients: Organic grass-fed buttermilk, water, curry leaves, mustard seeds, fenugreek seeds, ginger, salt, ice.

Directions: Mix ¼ cup of buttermilk with 1 cup of water and a pinch of salt. For the seasoning, heat 1 tsp of oil on a pan, and add mustard seeds, curry leaves, crushed ginger, and fenugreek seeds. Once they start crackling, add them to the buttermilk. Add ice and stir.

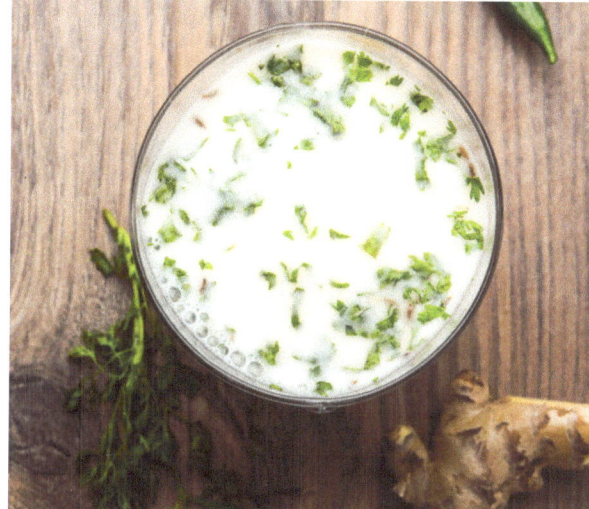

Neem cucumber lemon shots can help maintain healthy skin and lower blood sugar levels. However, excessive neem consumption can actually have the reverse effect, leading to hypoglycemia and indigestion. So, take it in small amounts and not more than twice a week. If the bitterness doesn't bother you, then an icy infusion of neem, cucumber and lemon can be quite refreshing!

Ingredients: Preservative-free neem juice, cucumber, lemon, rock salt, water

Directions: Blend 4 tbsp neem juice, ½ a cucumber, water, and salt. Add ice to the blended mixture and enjoy.

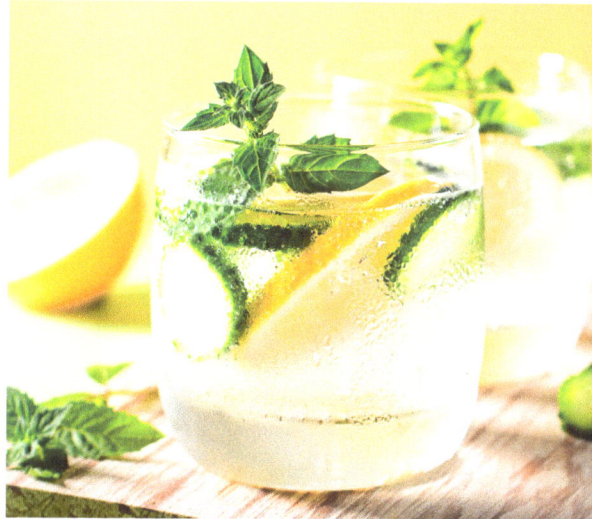

Bael (wood apple) or amla (gooseberry) sherbet is beneficial for weight loss, gastrointestinal problems, diabetes, and gynecological disorders, owing to the juices of these fruits. You can add some lemon juice and sweet mint leaves to avoid the bitter after-taste.

Ingredients: Fresh gooseberries or bael fruit (juice can also be store-bought)

Directions: Boil the fruit in water for 10 minutes. Once soft and warm, blend to make a pulp. Mix 2 tbsp of the pulp into 1 cup of water. Chill. Add fresh lemon juice, rock salt, and ice. Stir and enjoy!

None of the above drinks require added sugar. It's purely optional. These refreshing drinks will help maintain or reduce your blood sugar levels along with a good diet and exercise. They are best taken during the day and will satiate your cravings for sugary mocktails, juices, and shakes!

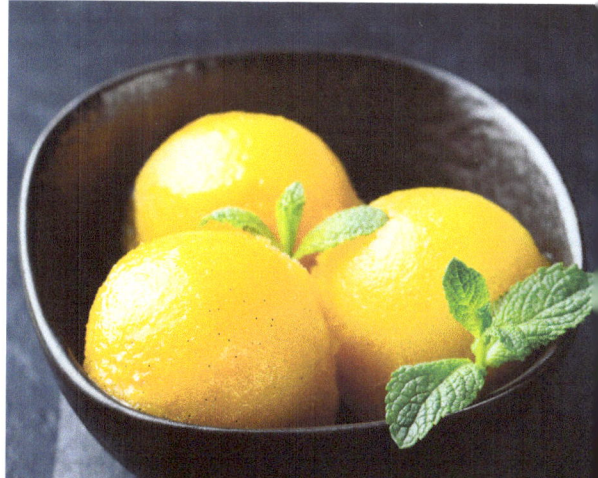